Preventing and Controlling Cancer in North America

Preventing and Controlling Cancer in North America

A Cross-Cultural Perspective

Edited by
Diane Weiner

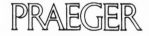

Westport, Connecticut
London

Library of Congress Cataloging-in-Publication Data

Preventing and controlling cancer in North America : a cross-cultural
    perspective / edited by Diane Weiner.
        p.   cm.
    Includes bibliographical references and index.
    ISBN 0–275–96180–X (alk. paper)
        1. Cancer—North America—Prevention—Cross-cultural studies.
    2. Health behavior—North America—Cross-cultural studies.
    I. Weiner, Diane (Diane E.)
    RC279.N58P74   1999
    362.1'96994'00973—dc21   99–19202

British Library Cataloguing in Publication Data is available.

Library of Congress Catalog Card Number: 99–19202
ISBN: 0–275–96180–X

First published in 1999

Praeger Publishers, 88 Post Road West, Westport, CT 06881
An imprint of Greenwood Publishing Group, Inc.
www.praeger.com

Printed in the United States of America

The paper used in this book complies with the
Permanent Paper Standard issued by the National
Information Standards Organization (Z39.48–1984).

10 9 8 7 6 5 4 3 2 1

Copyright Acknowledgments

The author and publisher gratefully acknowledge permission for use of the following material:

Chapter 3, "The Metastasis of Witchcraft: A Case Study of the Interrelationship between Traditional
and Biomedical Models," by Linda M. Hunt was originally published in *Collegium Antropologicum*
17, no. 2 (1993): 249–256.

This book is dedicated to the memory of Ramsey Ellis,
Computer Angel Extraordinaire (1981–1999)

Contents

PART III: *New Strategies for Cancer Research*

Illustrations

TABLES

FIGURES

Introduction

Jennie R. Joe

Each year, approximately 1.2 million people are diagnosed with cancer in the United States, and about seven million others are in remission (Chu and Krammer 1995). Included among the new cases diagnosed each year are individuals who are experiencing reoccurrence or second cancers. Much of what we know today indicates that most of these cancers could have been prevented (Ames et al. 1995).

With cancer among the leading causes of death for the U.S. population, the "war"on cancer marches at a steady pace, but perhaps with less fanfare than when President Richard Nixon signed the National Cancer Act in 1971 (Cairns 1985). While there has been considerable progress, the results of the cancer "war" thus far have been mixed. Clearly, one of the important successes has been in research, which has led to a better understanding of how cancer develops and progresses. Other cancer research and interventions have also helped lower mortality for certain cancer sites, although the decrease has not been equal for all segments of the American population. Those in the lower socioeconomic strata of society continue to have cancer mortality that is unchanged or, in some instances, has increased (Alexander 1995; Baquet and Hunter 1995). It should be noted, however, that breast and prostate cancers tend to be more prevalent among those of higher socioeconomic status (NCI 1998).

In addition to contributing to a greater understanding of the fundamentals of cancer cells, the "war" on cancer has also aided advancements in the care of individuals with cancer, that is, new modes of treatment and more effective treatment combinations or schedules. The undesirable side effects of therapy have also been decreased, and a reduction in surgical interventions has meant less pain, disfigurement, or loss of function for many cancer patients (Rennie and Rusting 1996).

Despite these advancements, however, cures for most cancers remain elusive, and other cancer-related issues, such as primary prevention, have not been fully addressed. A pressing need also remains for consistent and sufficient funding for cancer research, particularly initiatives that target special populations or minorities in clinical research and initiatives that help narrow the gap between the special populations and the rest of society in the rates of cancer survivorship (Warner 1995; NCI 1998).

In the mid 1980s, the disparity in health statistics between minority groups and the general population became a subject of concern at the national level. The attention was highlighted by an eight-volume report by the Task Force on Black and Minority Health (1985), a group commissioned by the United States Secretary of Health and Human Services. The report focused on a number of key problems that disproportionately affect the health status of the socioeconomically disadvantaged, a category that includes African Americans, Hispanics, Native Americans, and Asian Pacific Islanders. For these special populations, the discrepancies have resulted in shorter life expectancy, higher infant mortality, more birth defects, and a high prevalence of asthma, diabetes, cardiovascular disease, and cancer (DHHS 1985).

A year after the Task Force's reports were issued, the National Cancer Institute established a Special Populations Studies Branch within its Division of Cancer Prevention and Control. The Special Populations Branch was charged with a fourfold mission: (1) to plan, develop, implement, and evaluate a program of extramural intervention research targeting special populations (Hispanics, American Indians, Alaska Natives, Asians, and Pacific Islanders, African Americans, Native Hawaiians, blue-collar workers, rural, elderly, low-income, and low-literacy groups); (2) to identify barriers to prevention research; (3) to coordinate and maintain networks of researchers, health professionals, and community leaders in order to facilitate involvement in research of medically underserved populations; and (4) to develop a program to recruit individuals from "special populations" to pursue careers in research and to participate in research studies (NCI 1997a).

The Special Populations Branch initiated a number of key cancer research and training programs involving minorities, but it was quietly dismantled in 1996, when the National Cancer Institute created a new Office of Special Populations within the director's office. The stated purpose of the new program was to oversee the efforts of all the National Institutes of Health that target special populations. With coordination as its primary role, however, the new program did not inherit the resources or the authority to solicit or award the research or training grants that had been provided under the old program (NCI 1997a).

Poverty has been consistently identified as one of the most important and often recurring variables accounting for disparity in health status for the disadvantaged. Certain cancers that are disproportionately represented in special populations are often associated with low income; poverty particularly results in unhealthy lifestyles and behaviors and exposure to unhealthy environments. Tobacco smoking, high alcohol consumption, poor nutrition, and environmental exposure to certain carcinogens increase cancer risks for those who are socioeconomically disadvantaged. Researchers have also noted that although some of the difference in cancer morbidity and mortality between races may have a genetic basis, genetic differences are deemed to be greater *within* than among races (NCI 1986; DeVita et al. 1995; Bingham and Rull 1997).

Because there is strong evidence for the influence of behavioral factors in some cancer-incidence and mortality rates, the National Cancer Institute has directed considerable research effort toward modifying these risk behaviors. Some of the targeted areas have included smoking cessation, the development of the "5-A-Day" healthy eating paradigm, an emphasis on increased cancer screening, and a focus on behaviors that affect quality of life and prolong survival in the treatment of persons with cancer (NCI 1997b).

As laudable as these efforts are, the message has not reached all segments of society. Smoking, for example, has not decreased significantly among teens, women, or minorities. Women from minority and special populations also have less understanding of cancer risks and are less likely to follow breast and cervical cancer screening guidelines. Consequently, many members of these groups view all cancers as fatal or regard the disease with such fear that they resist any type of cancer screening. They "don't want to know" if they have cancer.

Culture also plays a major role in the perception of cancer and its prognosis; several differing sociocultural views and experiences with cancer are examined in this book. The authors present the perspectives of a variety of ethnic groups, with an emphasis on social, cultural, and behavioral aspects of the cancer experience. These ideas are grouped under three overarching themes: cancer beliefs and behaviors; interventions; and strategies for cancer research.

In the first chapter, Martha Balshem discusses selective events that have affected the historical patient-doctor relationship. The new, emerging relationship finds increasing numbers of patients questioning medical authority and a growing number of patients desiring to participate in medical decision making. The relationship has also been influenced by the growing acceptance of full disclosure when cancer is diagnosed. In this new patient-doctor relationship, Balshem observes, oncologists have difficulty in managing patients' false hopes or accepting the blame for treatment failures. These discussions and views of oncologists are placed within the context of the special patient-physician relationship that develops when a patient has cancer.

In the second chapter, David Hess reviews alternative and complementary cancer therapies (ACCTs) and their implications for cancer prevention and control. Hess attributes the growth of ACCTs to such factors as the increase in the cancer epidemic, growing patient dissatisfaction with traditional clinical treatments, poor long-term survival rates, and the influence of institutionalized alternative clinics in Mexico and Europe. Reviewing the development of ACCTs, Hess discusses the controversy regarding certain of these alternative therapies, both within and outside the circle of ACCT advocates.

Focusing on a young male bone cancer patient in Mexico, Chapter Three takes a look at the interrelationship between traditional and biomedical models. Linda Hunt examines various sociocultural implications of the diagnosis, not only for the patient but also for the family and the surrounding community. Hunt notes that in industrializing countries, like Mexico, biomedical recommendations regarding cancer treatments may be impossible to fulfill, because the resources are not accessible or the treatment is not affordable. In such cases, traditional treatment offered by the culture is the only alternative.

Chapter Four explores the theme of social support and the explicit or implicit influences of racial discrimination for African-American women with breast cancer. Rhonda Moore cites a study involving a sample of African-American women with breast cancer living in Houston, Texas, and the San Francisco Bay area. Excerpts from its interviews indicate that based on their personal experience, a number of the African-American women believe that cancer treatments favor white American women.

In Chapter Five, Diane Weiner examines the sociocultural perceptions of cancer through language, specifically through the mental image or fear that such words as "cancer" evoke in some American Indian tribal members. Among some southern California Indians, for example, cancer is thought to have multiple causes and death is not viewed as inevitable. Among other tribal groups, however, the occurrence of cancer may be attributed to evil thoughts and negativity. There is also the fear that because words sometimes have the power to cause things to happen, even talking about cancer can trigger it. Weiner cautions the reader that this sociocultural discourse on cancer is influenced by age, gender, and one's own experience with cancer survivors.

In Chapter Six, Ann Lanier and Janet Kelly present findings from the Alaska Native Women's Health Project, a research and service program that examined baseline knowledge, attitudes, and behaviors regarding cervical and breast cancer among a sample of Alaska Native women in Anchorage. The study sought to determine whether intervention changed or influenced the subjects' knowledge and cancer screening behaviors. One outcome of the study was an indication that the women did demonstrate greater knowledge about cancer risk after the intervention. The researchers also found, however, that women who were at high risk for cancer were unlikely either to score higher in cervical or breast cancer biomedical knowledge tests or be referred for cancer screening when they initially came into health facilities for other medical care needs.

Chapter Seven describes the development, implementation, and evaluation of a tobacco-use prevention and low-fat and high-fiber diet program designed for rural Native American children, their teachers, and their families. Sally M. Davis and Leslie Cunnignham-Sabo explore the different ways in which children learn in formal settings using a culturally specific curriculum that is guided by teachers and community role models. This unique project represents an approach in which academics, clinicians, educators, and community members cooperate in the creation and operation of youth-oriented cancer prevention programs within established institutions.

Chapter Eight assesses the effectiveness of utilizing physicians to encourage smoking cessation among a sample of African-American subjects. As part of the study, Bruce Allen and his colleagues developed a teaching protocol for physicians, who were given training in counseling patients to quit smoking. The outcome of the study suggested, however, that delivering smoking-cessation messages is not enough to motivate a smoker to quit.

In Chapter Nine, Bettye Green and Ellen Werner report the results of interviews with women who organized or directed breast cancer programs for African-American women in different parts of the United States. The programs varied from formal programs provided in university hospitals to informal approaches wherein volunteers led cancer survivor groups. Thoroughly describing the programs, the authors review factors that hampered or enriched the various approaches.

A culturally sensitive recruitment and retention model designed for use with Hispanic women in Texas is the subject of Chapter Ten. Lovell Jones and colleagues describe the unique aspects of the model, used to recruit and maintain Hispanic women in a nutrition clinical trial. One key aim in designing the model was to limit the study to a specific target group of Hispanic women, in order to identify and alleviate such potential barriers as language, accessibility, literacy levels, and cultural attitudes. Another objective was community representation throughout the project.

In Chapter Eleven, Judith Kaur suggests that cancer survivors might be ideal agents for social change. Using examples from Native American communities, Kaur notes that as change agents, cancer survivors not only support cancer patients and their families but also influence entire tribal communities' attitudes towards cancer. In support of this view, Kaur describes the workings of two such support groups, one in the Southwest (the Gathering of Cancer Support) and another in Alaska (the "Denaina Tee-Ya," which trains community health representatives to develop local support networks for cancer survivors in rural areas of the state).

Sociocultural aspects of breast cancer screening among Asian and Pacific Islander American women are discussed by Margie Kagawa-Singer and Annette E. Maxwell in Chapter Twelve. The authors note that among certain women, sociocultural perceptions of cancer, lack of knowledge, and the fear of breast cancer frequently present barriers to screening practices. The authors argue that beliefs about cancer etiologies also vary between and even within these groups, even though these groups are often aggregated for census, research, and health delivery purposes.

In Chapter Thirteen, Linda Burhansstipanov reviews issues that need to be addressed in order to improve the likelihood of developing and implementing culturally competent interventions. Citing as examples several programs for Native American communities, Burhansstipanov interprets a series of personal barriers, including more visible barriers (such as lack of transportation) and less visible ones (such as psychosocial factors). Based on several studies, she offers a variety of approaches to develop and operate culturally competent programs.

Chapter Fourteen raises the question of whether a relationship exists between physical activity and cancer in Hispanic populations. Lisa Staten notes that previous studies conducted on this question have been limited primarily to white Americans and the middle or upper socioeconomic strata of U. S. society. The author urges that Hispanics be included in future cancer research, particularly in view of national surveys

reporting that Hispanics are less active than white Americans. She also calls for validation of existing research instruments with this population.

Chapter Fifteen focuses on the role of diet in the promotion and suppression of cancer. Nicolette I. Teufel discusses diet-cancer associations and applies
them to dietary patterns and cancer incidence rates for Native Americans living in
the Southwest. One of Teufel's findings is that micronutrient intakes are often
greater than reported by many tribal members. Consumption of wild plant foods,
for example, may not be reported, because the most commonly used instrument,
the Food Frequency Questionnaire (FFQ), does not seek this information.

These chapters provide new information and fresh insights, and in all demonstrate vividly how differently cancer is viewed through these diverse cultural lenses.

LITERATURE CITED

Alexander, G. A. 1995. Cancer control in special populations: African-Americans, Native
    Americans, Hispanics, Poor and Underserved. In *Cancer prevention and control,*
    ed. P. Greenwald, B. S. Krammer, and D. L. Weed, 371–392. New York: Marcel
    Dekker.

Ames, B. N., L. Swirsky, and W. C. Willett. 1995. The causes and prevention of cancer.
    Proceedings of the National Academy of Sciences 92(12):5358–5365.

Baquet, C. R., and C. P. Hunter. 1995. Patterns in minorities and special populations. In
    Cancer prevention and control, ed. P. Greenwald, B. S. Krammer, and D. L.
    Weed, 23–36. New York: Marcel Dekker.

Bingham, E., and D. P. Rull. 1997. Preventive strategies for living in a chemical world: A
    symposium in honor of Irving J. Selikoff. *New York Academy of Science* 837.

Cairns, J. 1985. The treatment of disease and the war against cancer. *Scientific American*
    253(5):51–59.

Chu, K. C., and B. S. Krammer. 1995. Cancer patterns in the United States. In *Cancer
    prevention and control,* ed. P. Greenwald, B. S. Krammer, and D. L. Weed, 19–
    22. New York: Marcel Dekker.

DeVita, V. T. Jr., S. Hellman, and S. A. Rosenberg, eds. 1995. *Biological therapy of
    cancer.* 2nd ed. Philadelphia, PA: Lippincott.

Frank-Stromberg, M., and S. J. Olsen. 1993. *Cancer prevention in minority populations.* St.
    Louis, MO: Mosby.

The National Cancer Institute (NCI). 1986. *Cancer among black and other minorities: A
    statistical profile.* Bethesda, MD: National Institutes of Health. National Cancer
    Institute.

—. 1997a. Focus research efforts on underserved populations and those with a dispropor-
    tionate cancer burden. Unpublished report of the Cancer Control Program Review
    Group. Bethesda, MD: National Cancer Institute, September 15.

—. 1997b. Behavioral research and behavioral interventions trials in cancer prevention.
    Unpublished director's report on the Cancer Prevention Program. Bethesda, MD:
    National Cancer Institute, June 13.

—. 1998. *The nation's investment in cancer research.* Bethesda, MD: National Institutes of
    Health. National Cancer Institute.

Rennie, J., and R. Rusting. 1996. Making headway against cancer. *Scientific American*
    274(3):56–59.

US DHHS. 1985. *Report of the secretary's task force on black and minority health.* Washington, DC: Department of Health and Human Services.

Warner, K. E. 1995. Public policy issues. In *Cancer prevention and control,* ed. P. Green-wald, B. S. Kramer, and D. L. Weed, 451–472. New York: Mercel Dekker.

Part I

Cancer Beliefs and Behaviors

Chapter 1

Negotiating Medical Authority: Contradictions in Oncology Practice

Martha Balshem

INTRODUCTION

Scientific medicine is a fascinating system. It is easy to get lost in its minutiae, to forget to see how the lifeworld (Mishler et al. 1981) fashions the life of the clinic, and to portray physicians as disembodied representatives of rational medical perspectives. Sometimes we miss how the irrational in physician experience—history, emotional need, construction of self, yearnings for transcendent meaning—shapes medical practice.

The circumstances of practice in oncology make it difficult to miss the emotion in the physician. In oncology, patients die, physicians weep, and wrenching loss is part of the ebb and flow of clinic life. Recent social anthropology in the cancer clinic has explored this emotional and cultural complexity. DelVecchio Good et al. (1990) review Italian, Japanese, and American disclosure of cancer diagnosis and examine the struggles of American oncologists, who attempt simultaneously to disclose openly, instill hope in patients, and maintain their own sense of optimism about treatment. Hunt (1992) explores the complex interrelationships between medical authority, class authority, and styles of disclosure in a Mexican clinic. Balshem (1993) describes the sometimes irresolvable conflict that can arise when oncologist and family hold competing versions of a cancer death. DelVecchio Good et al. (1994) describe how oncologists attempt to guide their patients between false hope and despair, always favoring immediacy over troubling questions about the future.

As this literature shows, practice in medical oncology is fraught with dilemmas and contradictions. Here I examine contradictions in authority experienced by medical oncologists in the United States and look for synchronicities (Jackson 1989) between clinic and lifeworld. Like the literature cited above, my analysis is relevant to medical practice in many fields. In the oncology clinic, however, physicians and patients deal with life-threatening illness; thus, emotion and cultural contradiction are especially visible.

My analysis is based on approximately seventy hours of clinical observation. Informal discussions with oncologists, oncology nurses, physician's assistants, counselors, medical assistants, and patients occurred during the course of these observations. I also conducted formal ethnographic interviews with ten oncologists; these interviews, lasting an average of an hour, were guided by a brief list of open-ended questions focused on the emotional aspects of oncology practice. In addition, I have drawn on insights developed during my three and a half years of employment in cancer prevention research at a major comprehensive cancer center.

A BRIEF HISTORY

In his social history of cancer in the United States, Patterson (1987) describes the coalition formed in the late nineteenth and early twentieth centuries between practitioners of scientific medicine, who were consolidating their social and legal supremacy in American medicine, and social activists from the same upper-class milieu. Together, they raised and publicized the hope that science could cure cancer. The political skills of this coalition were such that in 1938 Congress created the National Cancer Institute (NCI), the first, and still the biggest, of the National Institutes of Health. Government zeal to fund cancer research was disproportionately great compared with research success. Nevertheless, following World War II NCI budgets boomed, along with public confidence in the power of science to cure all our ills.

The first major advances in cancer therapy—chemotherapy for the treatment of leukemias and lymphomas—were made in the 1940s and 1950s. In 1954, the American Cancer Society (ACS) released the first major study showing that smoking causes cancer. These developments encouraged the popular perception that science was making great progress against cancer and would certainly soon find a cure. Environmental theories regarding cancer causation were pushed aside as medical scientists and the lay public alike became fascinated with cellular mechanisms, a fascination that promoted and was promoted by a focus on the individual body. Hope and faith were high. At the same time, cancerphobia was still strong, among both lay people and physicians. As late as 1961, 90% of the physicians of one hospital stated that they usually did not inform a patient of a diagnosis of cancer (Oken 1961. This study was critical of such practice.)

By the late 1960s and early 1970s, cancer research had progressed on numerous fronts, with new knowledge about the carcinogenicity of various chemicals, the possible involvement of viral agents in carcinogenesis, the links between hormones and cancer, the workings of the immune system, the specifics of metastatic processes, the epidemiology of cancer and occupation, and the links between cancer and diet (Raven 1985). In 1964, the Surgeon General's report on smoking and cancer was issued; limitations on cigarette advertising followed. The time was ripe for the birth of oncology, a new medical specialty. Chemotherapy was now being used to treat solid tumors, and knowledge about treating cancers was growing. This supported specialization among both physicians and nurses (Blume 1991). Professional attitudes towards cancer care changed as well. By 1970, physicians in one small community hospital had shifted toward more frequent disclosure of the diagnosis of cancer, probably reflecting a growing feeling that some effective therapies for cancer did exist (Friedman 1970).

The optimism of the times infected physicians involved in devising new strategies for cancer treatment. These new specialists felt like medical pioneers: one of my interview subjects, for example, was for a time the only physician in a sizable metropolitan area with special training in oncology. In 1971, President Richard Nixon signed the National Cancer Act, speaking in stirring words about the "war against cancer." For the next four years, the budget of the NCI increased faster than the rate of inflation (Yarbro 1985) and provided funding for fellowships in oncology and hematology. The American Board of Internal Medicine established these two fields as subspecialties, giving the first board examination in hematology in 1972 and the first examination in oncology in 1973.[1]

Just at this bright beginning, however, public optimism about cancer science began to sour. The 1960s and early 1970s were a time of upheaval in the United States. Following the civil rights movement, ever-widening sectors of the population of the United States mobilized to challenge various social and political authorities. It was a time in which social power and the boundaries of social roles became more negotiable and flexible (Martin 1994). People in medical school or preparing to enter medical school were affected by this, and some joined organizations concerned with the social reform of medicine.

In the context of the general loss of faith in authority that deepened through the post-Vietnam, post-Watergate era, patients became "medical consumers," prepared to challenge physicians and make decisions about their own care (Reeder 1972). In this context, the general public turned a suspicious eye at cancer care and cancer science. The growing environmental movement gave enormous impetus to what Patterson calls the "cancer counterculture." A spate of books and articles took the "cancer establishment" to task: criticizing individualist theories of cancer causation as blaming the victim; accusing the ACS and NCI of slighting cancer prevention; claiming a cover-up of the environmental causes of cancer, particularly workplace hazards and hazards from pollution; and blaming proprietorial greed of establishment medical institutions for denying public access to such unorthodox cancer treatments as Laetrile. Much of the cancer counterculture literature was marred by careless arguments, hostile assertions, and loosely framed conspiracy theories. The sound criticisms that appeared also emerged in the mainstream medical literature. Many mainstream analysts, for instance, feel that funding for cancer prevention and attention to the subject in oncology training and conferences is inadequate (Meyskens 1988; Heimendinger et al. 1990). In any case, the popularity of the cancer counterculture literature was (and is) based on a keenly felt distrust of mainstream medical authority.

The field of oncology, then, was born into a contradiction. On one hand, oncology is a child of post–World War II confidence in science and medicine. This spirit still animates the field: many oncologists in practice today remember when the field was pioneered, much of its science and medicine is very new, most oncologists have patients enrolled in clinical trials, and fellows in oncology still spend more time in research than those in most other fields (Lyttle et al. 1991). Oncologists are still excited about applying science at the bedside—and see theirs as the most exciting science in medicine or basic biology.[2]

On the other hand, oncology is the child of a collapse of faith in medical authority. Oncology patients demand participation in medical decision making, and they pressure physicians toward more personal and egalitarian relationships. Dying patients request higher social status, supported by death-and-dying studies that have criticized physicians and others for anticipatory withdrawal from dying people (Novack et al. 1979). This has all had a formative influence on oncology, complicating and contradicting the oncologist's heritage of optimism about exerting the authority of medicine.

In the two oncology clinics I observed, oncologists struggled with this contradiction on a daily basis. Their struggles were easy to see in their disclosure practices. In most national and traditional medical systems, a diagnosis of cancer is kept secret from most patients. In the United States, however, full disclosure of cancer diagnosis to almost all patients is an ideal of practice.[3] In one sense, this is aggressive medicine—or perhaps aggressive medical authority—based on an aggressive faith in cancer treatment. In another sense, it is based on the patient's right to know and participate in decision making about treatment. In either case, negotiations between oncologists and their patients regarding medical authority are right up front for the social analyst to see.

THE BURDENS OF HOPE AND ANGER

There are several issues that make medical authority especially hard for oncologists to negotiate. One such issue is that of "false hope." In every case thought of as terminal, the moment comes when the oncologist needs the patient to understand the imminence of death. For the oncologist to deal with this moment effectively, the patient must cooperate and signal an understanding of the necessity to give up hope. Not every patient will do this. The following quotations from three medical oncologists show the physician's angst when the patient holds onto hope that the physician sees as unrealistic:

I'm gonna see a patient on Friday. She's only 38. *She's* dying of breast cancer. *I* have to tell her that her MRI scan was worse. What I want her to do, is to say, "Gee, doc, I'm gonna die, I guess I have to accept it." 'Cause that'll make *me* feel like a—not so bad. She's not gonna do that. She's going to get all upset and she's gonna say, "What do I do now to *beat* this thing." And *I know* she can't, but *she* doesn't know it, and *how* am I gonna deal with that? . . . So *one possible* reaction is to get angry at *her* for not accepting the inevitable.

To try and convey to people what the situation is objectively, in a manner that they can understand, I think is probably about the most challenging thing. . . . To some people it may be important to just keep tilting at windmills until the day they die, but . . . I think that those people are much more likely to compromise their remaining time than they are to enhance their remaining time. So that, to me, goes against the basic idea of [oncology practice], which is helping cancer patients whether you're treating their cancer or not.

One of the things I have almost no trouble with feeling negative about at all is patients refusing treatment. . . . I have more difficulty sometimes with patients where they want to be treated to the last moment, to the last dying breath. And I want desperately just to let these people go into hospice, but they won't do it.

The patient who wants to be treated "to the last dying breath" may claim to feel "thrilled" at failing a standard chemotherapy course, because that opens the way to another, stronger drug that will "surely bring about a cure." Such a patient might seek treatments publicized in the news media and refuse to believe that treatment options are exhausted. Faced with this, oncologists cannot negotiate their own needs: aggressive medical authority fails, and so does shared decision making.

Accusatory patients pose similar problems. Such patients blame the oncologist for the failure of treatment or for the patient's imminent death. Such a patient refuses ownership of his or her own death and pushes ownership onto the oncologist instead. I would have lived, the narrative goes, but you did something wrong. Sometimes family members continue this narrative after the patient's death. These oncologists speak about living with anger and accusation:

Either the patient or the family is angry about cancer. And they—they don't want to blame themselves, so they have to blame someone. Now, the patient can't blame his wife, that's not fair, um, let's blame the health professionals. And not—and it doesn't come out, in the sense, you—you're responsible for *my* getting cancer, but—why can't you cure me? You know, the physician is angry, he *can't* cure someone. And who did *that* anger get transferred to? You know, it—you don't want to transfer it to the patient, cause you feel so bad for them, so maybe you'll transfer it to the family. You know, *why can't you work* with me to help this patient?

It does make you angry. I had an experience a couple of weeks ago, a woman who has advanced breast cancer, and had basically an hour's worth of reasons that she had come up with about why she wasn't doing well. And all of them were assigning blame to a lot of people along the way, and I was a major component in that. You know, supposedly not giving her her drug on time, and not allowing this to happen and not allowing that to happen. We spent the better part of an hour going over her chart and going over records and just attempting to give her a database that would crack through her misconceptions, and trying to do that in a non-critical way. But inside it made me furious, and I have no illusion that that didn't show a bit.

I guess the hardest type of patient is one who comes in and is angry. And the anger prevents them from—first of all, from letting us take care of them. . . . The oncology unit gets a lot of anger. . . . Those are the most frustrating in that the first thing you want to do is kick them and boot them out. To say, "Well, okay, if you don't want me to help you, fine, then get out of here." But on the other hand, they're the biggest challenge. A lot of that is that they're angry at you, but not you as a person. They're angry at you as a representative of telling them what they have.

These oncologists live with their own anger toward the accusatory patient, with whom they can negotiate neither respect for medical authority nor any form of consensus.

THE GOOD DEATH

As a patient's death approaches, the contradictions in the oncologist's practice take a turn. Aggressive medical authority ceases to be relevant; it is time to cede authority to the patient. The ideal patient accepts the oncologist's pronouncement that treatment has come to an end. The patient puts his or her affairs in order, leaves nothing unsaid, and accepts the recommended palliative care. Such a death the oncologist can accept—she or he has ushered in a good death. Some patients, however, do not follow the ideal pattern and prevent the oncologist from feeling like an ideal physician. Oncologists may feel that they have failed not only if the patient dies but also if the patient does not die well. The following statements illustrate this:

He would have died, anyway, but still, I think it's important to give a family a good death. I mean, that sounds a little crude, but—like giving a mother a good birth, it's not just the baby that counts, it's the experience, her whole ability to handle that experience. I think the same thing is true on the other end of life.

In medicine, we're expected to make people better and to help them and heal them if you can, or get them to feel better. So there's a good part of me that just sort of figures that is expected of me. In medicine, you're taught to be sort of self-accusatory, you know, for making mistakes. But I'd say that you have to look for the up sides, too. I think that it's participating in something that's meaningful, like even helping somebody to die. That may be not a down thing if you do a good job of it.

Most people who are going to be in oncology are going to be people that personally have somewhere along the line come to some personal philosophy and acceptance—I don't know what the right word is—of death. If you were in this field and every time you have death you felt that that was a failure, it would be an extraordinarily frustrating field. So you have to have a philosophy that says, I'm here to help a person and their family have the best-quality adjustment to this disease process as possible. And yes, someone may die. The rest of the family goes on living, however, and they need to come out the other side, somehow, not broken.

Residents being socialized into oncology practice are exposed to these ways of thinking. The following bears on this:

That, by the way, that's a very difficult thing to teach our residents. It's one of our biggest sources of conflict between the oncologist and the resident. Most of these residents aren't going to be oncologists. They're only at the internal medicine stage. They want to be, "This patient's going to die, let's stop the I.V.s today, why futz around?" They don't understand the process or the time it takes for either a patient or a family to absorb certain things. It's the biggest source of frustration. Whenever I attend on the ward, there's always at least one or two incidents a month where the residents get very upset. They think we're torturing the patient. They think we're causing their life to be prolonged unnecessarily just because [a family member] can't make a decision. They identify very much with the patient. They want the patient to be comfortable, and if that means dead, you know, if that's the only way—and sometimes the other [family] members involved aren't quite ready to take that step. It's hard to kind of hold [the residents'] hands through it and assure them it really will happen. You know, we're really not being cruel.

Here, the oncologist assumes responsibility even as medical authority gives way to accepting the patient's authority over his or her own death. Patients have the right to die as they wish—to see their charts, disagree with the physician, get a second opinion, and make decisions for themselves. Oncologists I worked with feel with conviction—feel it as an ethical issue—that patients have the right to be ready for death, to decide when to take risks with death or whether or not to fight it. The following illustrates this ideal of practice:

It has evolved over the last several years that the physician's role is as an advisor, not as a guide, and our job now is to tell people what can be done. What the pros, what the cons, what the good, what the bad. And I openly tell every one of my chemotherapy patients, you are going to make the final decisions on what's done. And what we're going to do is talk about what can be done. I say, if I don't agree with your decision, I may argue with you, you know, but the final decision is going to be yours. It wasn't true twenty years ago. People came in and they were told, this is what you're going to do.

However, many oncologists do assume emotional responsibility beyond the time for aggressive medicine, into the time for the patient's negotiation with death. For the oncologist to negotiate the contradictions of practice, both must be done right.

"Nobody lies. That's the first rule," said one medical assistant of life in her clinic. This ethic, deeply felt by many oncologists practicing in the United States, makes great emotional demands on oncologists and patients alike, but if open disclosure can be negotiated successfully, there are great rewards for them both. Most patients do, in fact, live out the above-described image of ideal behavior in dying or living with cancer. Thus, the oncologist has more occasion to be gratified and inspired than depressed and frustrated.

On one occasion, after I watched an oncologist and a patient discussing the course of the patient's disease, I asked the oncologist if it had been a difficult discussion, considering that the patient was dying. The oncologist was affronted: "She's *very much alive!*" he said. He then insisted that I follow him to his office, where he rummaged through his files and found a research paper showing a mortality curve for the patient's disease. According to the curve, the patient's life expectancy was indeed very short; however, she had already survived much longer than expected. With treatment, he said, he had given her time, good quality time. His faith and aggressive optimism were clear; so were his advocacy of and admiration for the patient. I imagined the future: he would treat with optimism as long as he could; he would cede his authority to her when the time came; he would find his own sense of peace if the time, and her decisions, seemed right to him.

CONCLUSION

Practice in medical oncology involves constant negotiation. Oncologists and patients negotiate about who is in charge, and oncologists negotiate a path between the exercise of authority and respect for patient autonomy. In this, oncologists do not differ from other physicians who work with patients: the contradictions described here affect the patient-physician relationship in most fields. In oncology, however, because cancer is life-threatening, the negotiations are present in stark relief.

For many of the oncologists whose practice I observed, the key to successful negotiation seemed to lie in the emotional bonds between oncologist and patient. In both clinics I observed, there were also strong emotional bonds among staff members, including the oncologists. People shared each other's grief, attended funerals together, and supported each other with humor and affection. Whatever the clinic environment, oncologists and their patients must negotiate life-shattering experiences together. During the usually long courses of treatment, they often get to know each other well. Oncology patients need this support, but the oncologists I observed seemed to need it too. Among the oncologists I interviewed, one spoke most movingly of this:

Having done the bone marrow, you sit down on the bed or wherever the person is, and actually describe the fact that they have leukemia. I would say that at those times you are as close to life and death at those minutes—maybe not death, but you're certainly close to something, something real deep. It's just something real deep in the spirit, I think, that you have, when you are able to have the privilege of seeing somebody like that and talking to them and experiencing—in my experience, anyhow, such an up-welling of deep courage, sometimes, and such deep inner beauty . . . and then the very next words out of my mouth will be, and we have some plans and we'll just walk down the road together and take it together. And then I think they feel like they have some company coming down the way. . . . It is a privilege, because of the depth of what is happening at those times. You know, how do you say the words? The life stories go before the patient's eyes. Here you're telling them something— and so I think you feel the impact of that. And you're sort of standing in awe of that—of— ah, I don't know, one's love of life. I'm not talking about life on a superficial level, I'm talking about life on a deep level, which a lot of us don't lead very often.

Cancer poses powerful contradictions: fighting death and accepting death, faith in medical authority and the ending of that faith. In the end, oncologists can sometimes resolve these contradictions in emotional bonds with their patients. Open disclosure creates a space where this is possible. Within this space, contradictions can dissolve; where there is affection and agreement, issues of authority fade; where talk bridges the gap between patient and oncologist, oncologists can feel a sense of privilege in their work. There is synchronicity here with the American impulse to seek healing in talk—in this case, to heal both oncologist and patient from the exercise of medical authority. Oncologists and their patients can negotiate medical authority together. If they are successful, the oncologist can escape, perhaps, from the contradictions of assuming medical authority in a postmodern world.

ACKNOWLEDGMENTS

I would like to thank the physicians, physician's assistants, medical assistants, nurses, and social workers who welcomed me into their workplaces and granted me interviews, and the patients who allowed me to observe their clinic appointments and chat with them while they underwent various procedures. I am very grateful to Ivan Karp, Mary-Jo DelVecchio Good, and Diane Weiner for comments on earlier versions of this paper.

NOTES

1.   Administratively, oncology is actually a subspecialty of internal medicine. Hematology is a closely related subspecialty. Training in the two subspecialties is often combined.

2.   Funding for basic cancer research is no longer as ample as it once was. This is partly a result of decreased funding for research and social programs, and partly, in the case of the National Cancer Institute, to an increase in funding for AIDS research (Korn 1989; Kerkvliet 1990). However, it is still possible for medical oncologists to maintain high research involvement through clinical trials, and many do.

3.   The movement toward full disclosure, rooted in the late 1960s, became a landslide in the 1970s. In a 1977 study of one group of hospital-based physicians, 98% reported that they generally did disclose a cancer diagnosis, and 100% reported that they would want to be told if they had cancer (Novack et al. 1979; compare to Oken 1961, in which only 60% of physicians stated that they would want to be told). Open disclosure, of course, is an ideal that appears neater in cultural analysis than it does in actual practice (see DiGiacomo 1987 for a description of an inadequate and contested disclosure process). Many practitioners in other national traditions see open disclosure, even when well handled, as cruel or as favoring patient autonomy too strongly over the principle of medical beneficence (Dalla-Vorgia et al. 1992; Pellegrino 1992; Surbone 1992, 1993; Capone 1993; Daly 1993; Lear 1993; Liberati 1993; Siegal 1993; Thomsen et al. 1993). Even in the United States, oncologists may wonder, in the words of one of my informants, "what we are accomplishing by all this telling" (see Holland 1989 for a discussion.)

LITERATURE CITED

Balshem, Martha. 1993. *Cancer in the community.* Washington, DC: Smithsonian Institution Press.

Blume, Elaine. 1991. Oncology professions transformed in 20 years: Patients benefit. *Journal of the National Cancer Institute* 83(9):596–598.

Capone, Ralph A. 1993. Letter. *Journal of the American Medical Association* 269(8):988–989.

Dalla-Vorgia, P., K. Katsouyanni, T. N. Garanis, G. Touloumi, P. Drogari, and A. Koutselinis. 1992. Attitudes of a Mediterranean population to the truth-telling issue. *Journal of Medical Ethics* 18:67–74.

Daly, Mary B. 1993. Letter. *New York Times Magazine*, February 14:8.

DelVecchio Good, Mary-Jo, Byron J. Good, Cynthia Schaffer, and Stuart E. Lind. 1990. American oncology and the discourse on hope. *Culture, Medicine, and Psychiatry* 14(1):59–79.

DelVecchio Good, Mary-Jo, Tseunetsugu Munakata, Yasuki Kobayashi, Cheryl Mattingly, and Byron J. G. 1994. Oncology and narrative time. *Social Science and Medicine* 38(6):855–862.

DiGiacomo, Susan M. 1987. Biomedicine as a cultural system: An anthropologist in the kingdom of the sick. In *Encounters with biomedicine: Case studies in medical anthropology*, ed. Hans A. Baer, 315–346. Philadelphia: Gordon and Breach Science Publishers.

Friedman, Henry J. 1970. Physician management of dying patients: An exploration. *Psychiatry in Medicine* 1:295–305.

Heimendinger, Jerianne, Susan Foerster, Mildred Kaufman, and Luise Light. 1990. Nutrition and cancer prevention activities in state health agencies. *Health Education Research* 5(4):545–550.

Holland, Jimmie C. 1989. Now we tell—but how well? *Journal of Clinical Oncology* 7(5):557–559.

Hunt, Linda. 1992. *Living with cancer in Oaxaca, Mexico: Patient and physician perspectives in cultural context.* Ph.D. dissertation, Harvard University.

Jackson, Michael. 1989. *Paths toward a clearing: Radical empiricism and ethnographic inquiry.* Bloomington: Indiana University Press.

Kerkvliet, Gary J. 1990. What's going on with research project grant funding at NCI? *Journal of the National Cancer Institute* 82(10):810–812.

Korn, David. 1989. Funding for cancer centers: A challenge of scarce resource allocation. *Journal of the National Cancer Institute* 81(24):1870–1873.

Lear, Martha Weinman. 1993. Should doctors tell the truth? The case against terminal candor. *New York Times Magazine*, January 24:17.

Liberati, Alessandro, Paula Mosconi, and Beth Meyerowitz. 1993. Letter. *Journal of the American Medical Association* 269(8):989.

Lyttle, Christopher S., Ronald M. Andersen, Kristen Neymarc, Christian Schmidt, Claire H. Kohrman, and Gerald S. Levey. 1991. National study of internal medicine manpower XVIII: Subspecialty fellowships with a special look at hematology and oncology, 1988–1989. *Annals of Internal Medicine* 114(1):36–42.

Martin, Emily. 1994. *Flexible bodies: Tracking Immunity in American culture—from the days of polio to the age of AIDS.* Boston: Beacon.

Meyskens, Frank L., Jr. 1988. Rethinking medical oncology training and education, Letter. *Journal of Clinical Oncology* 6(3):561–562.

Mishler, Elliot G., Lorna R. Amarasingham, Stuart T. Hauser, Ramsay Liem, Samuel D. Osherson, and Nancy E. Waxler. 1981. *Social contexts of health, illness, and patient care.* Cambridge, England: Cambridge University Press.

Novack, Dennis H., Robin Plumer, Raymond L. Smith, Herbert Ochitill, Gary R. Morrow, and John M. Bennett. 1979. Changes in physicians' attitudes toward telling the cancer patient. *Journal of the American Medical Association* 241(9):897–900.

Oken, Donald. 1961. What to tell cancer patients: A study of medical attitudes. *Journal of the American Medical Association* 175:1120–1128.

Patterson, James T. 1987. *The dread disease: Cancer and modern American culture.* Cambridge, MA: Harvard University Press.

Pellegrino, Edmund. 1992. Is truth telling to the patient a cultural artifact? *Journal of the American Medical Association* 268(13):1734–1735.

Raven, Ronald W. 1985. The development and practice of oncology. In *Cancer treatment and research in humanistic perspective*, ed. Steven C. Gross and Solomon Garb, 65–79. New York: Springer.

Reeder, Leo G. 1972. The patient-client as a consumer: Some observations on the changing professional-client relationship. *Journal of Health and Social Behavior* 13(4):406–412.

Siegal, Bernie S. 1993. Letter. *New York Times Magazine*, February 14:8.

Surbone, Antonella. 1992. Truth telling to the patient. *Journal of the American Medical Association* 268(13):1661–1662.

—. 1993. Letter. *Journal of the American Medical Association* 269(8):989.

Thomsen, Ole Ostergaard, Henrik R. Wulff, Alessandro Martin, and Peter A. Singer. 1993. What do gastroenterologists in Europe tell cancer patients? *Lancet* 341:473–476.

Yarbro, J. W. 1985. Cancer research and the development of cancer centers. In *Cancer Treatment and Research in Humanistic Perspective*, ed. Steven C. Gross and Solomon Garb, 3-15. New York: Springer.

Chapter 2

Patients, Science, and Alternative Cancer Therapies

David J. Hess

The percentage of the U.S. population that was expected to develop invasive cancer at some point in their lifetime was 38% for women and 48% for men in the 1991–1993 period (Parker et al. 1997). Another way of expressing the magnitude of the cancer epidemic is that one and a quarter million persons in the United States are diagnosed with cancer per year, and another 800,000 persons are diagnosed with basal cell and squamous cell skin cancers. About half a million people die from cancer each year, making the disease the second leading cause of death.

The problem is not solely one of magnitude: conventional therapies have an unsatisfactory track record. Five-year survival rates have remained largely static during the decades subsequent to President Richard Nixon's declaration of the war on cancer. As pathologist and environmental cancer expert Samuel Epstein comments,

According to the NCI's [National Cancer Institute's] own statistics, overall five-year survival rates for cancers in all ages and races improved marginally from 49.1% to 51.1% from 1974 to 1987—the rates for African Americans during this period actually dropped from 38.6% to 38.4%. Even this minuscule improvement in overall "cure" rates may be little more than statistical artifact: earlier diagnosis, for example, may extend the period between diagnosis and death, leading to the conclusion that the patient has survived longer, when the cancer may have proved fatal regardless of when it was diagnosed (1992, 234).

Likewise, according to veteran cancer activist and researcher Ralph Moss, the list of cancers responsive to chemotherapy was almost the same in the 1990s as in 1971, notwithstanding a quarter-century of research and the expenditure of tens of billions of dollars on research (1995, 81).

Given the dismal picture in terms of the size of the cancer epidemic and the poor chances for long-term survival that many cancer patients face, it is not surprising that they have turned to various alternative and complementary cancer therapies (ACCTs). An often-quoted survey in the *New England Journal of Medicine* suggests that more than 34% of the American people had resorted to at least one unconventional therapy during the year prior to the survey (Eisenberg et al. 1993). Estimates for the use of alternative therapies for cancer in the United States run from 10 to 50% of cancer patients; even the conservative end of the estimates suggests that at minimum the number of cancer patients in this category is probably between half a million and a million people (McGinnis 1991). Survey data suggest that users of ACCTs tend to be better educated than the population as a whole (Cassileth et al. 1984; Sharma 1992; Furnham and Forey 1994), although the data do not take into account variations within the population that might be associated with linkages between ethnic groups and traditional ethnic medicine. It is therefore likely that as the population becomes more educated about treatment options, cancer patients will tend to use more alternative and complementary therapies. As the number of patients using ACCTs grows, their views will have an increasing impact on regulatory policy and research agendas. This study will describe some of the major contours of the ACCT movement in the United States and their implications for the prevention and control of cancer in North America.

BACKGROUND

Let us estimate that over one million Americans are using ACCTs in some way for the treatment of cancer. Probably the bulk of those patients could be described as minimal users of complementary therapies. The use of the term "complementary" raises the vexed issue of the politics of terminology. A number of charged terms, such as "quack," "unproven," "questionable," and "unconventional" therapies, appear in the literature, usually employed by persons who do not have adequate credentials in the social sciences and have no interest in developing an accurate portrayal of the ACCT movement as a social phenomenon. Likewise, the idea that there is "no alternative medicine, only medical alternatives," which one sometimes hears from opponents of ACCTs, suggests a political naivete, which this chapter will question. The terminology is therefore highly charged and warrants some clarification.

I use the terms "alternative" and "complementary" as sociocultural descriptors of differences in usage patterns. The term "alternative" denotes a usage in place of such conventional therapies as surgery, radiation, and chemotherapy; "complementary" denotes usage alongside conventional therapies as adjuvants (British Medical Association 1993). The same therapeutic intervention, such as vitamin C, can be either alternative or complementary, depending on how it is used. It is probable that the bulk of patients who might be classified as users of ACCTs are using them as complementary interventions. For example, instead of taking high doses of intravenous vitamin C infusions as part of an alternative protocol, most patients are probably taking some oral supplement as an adjuvant to conventional methods.

The group of therapies in the ACCT range can be classified in different ways. In readings and conferences, the following categories were used: psycho-spiritual interventions, dietary programs, supplements, nontoxic pharmacological and immunological modalities, and herbs. Many of the psychospiritual interventions, such as group psychotherapy, have now achieved acceptance in the medical community as valuable adjunctive therapies. Some aspects of dietary programs, supplements, and herbs have also been integrated into conventional protocols in hospitals in the United States, again as adjunctive therapies. However, when those modalities are combined and offered as alternatives to conventional therapies, they remain controversial. Likewise, the nontoxic pharmacological and immunological modalities tend to be offered as alternatives and to be highly controversial. Those modalities include immunotherapies (such as bacterial vaccines), peptides (known as antineoplastons), blood fractions (known as immuno-augmentative therapy), a nontoxic chemotherapeutic substance (known as laetrile), oxygen therapies such as ozone and hydrogen peroxide, and a product designed to control cachexia (known as hydrazine sulfate).

The research presented herein is based on interviews with opinion leaders of the ACCT movement. Those interviews are broken down into two groups of roughly equivalent size. The first group includes about two dozen of the leading clinicians, researchers, journalists, and heads of information-providing organizations. The interviews in this group are the topic of a book (Hess 1999). The second group involves women patients, mostly breast cancer patients, who have used ACCTs and have subsequently become involved as leaders of the movement to open up medical treatments for women cancer patients. Most of the women have written books on the topic; others have volunteered as workers in patient support organizations. The interviews in this group and discussion of general themes and policy issues were published in the book *Women Confront Cancer* (Wooddell and Hess 1998) and will not be discussed here.

THE STRUCTURE OF THE ALTERNATIVE CANCER THERAPY MOVEMENT

The ACCT movement today in North America has changed dramatically since the 1970s. Social science reports of the ACCT movement of the 1970s described the political mobilization surrounding laetrile and the divisions within the movement, between groups associated with right-wing politics and those with a more liberal or left-wing political orientation (e.g., Peterson and Markle 1979a, 1979b). Today, the ACCT movement is much more diverse, both in terms of the number of major organizations involved and the number of therapies offered.

Although there are no adequate quantitative measures of the growth of the ACCT movement, the number of publications, institutions, clinicians, and patient support organizations has grown substantially since the 1970s. Several background social changes suggest that the pattern of growth is long-term and systemic:

1.   the globalization of medical care through the institutionalization of alternative clinics in Mexico and Europe, and the movement of thousands of patients per year

across international borders, such that a de facto deregulation has occurred as a result of globalization;

2. the growth of health maintenance organizations that are beginning to accept less-expensive alternative therapies in response to cost-benefit analysis and patient demand (although funding for ACCTs may prove much more difficult to achieve than for other chronic diseases and conditions);

3. the widespread dissemination of information through decentralized mass media (health-food books, small magazines, direct mail campaigns, and the Internet); and

4. the growth and professionalization of such alternative health care providers as naturopaths and specialists in Chinese traditional medicine.

In addition, epidemiological data suggest that age-standardized incidence rates have climbed steadily at a rate of about 1% per year, at least until recently; thus there has been a long-term increase in the patient population in the United States (Davis et al. 1994, 431).

American patients who pursue ACCTs are sometimes able to find a medical doctor, naturopathic doctor, or other health-care provider who is willing to supervise the case locally. However, each year thousands also go to foreign clinics and hospitals. The best known are the Lukas and Janker clinics in central Europe, the immuno-augmentative therapy (Burton) clinic in the Bahamas, and the dozens of clinics and hospitals in Mexico, principally Tijuana. The growth of ACCTs in Tijuana has been phenomenal, from just a few clinics in the early 1970s to over thirty clinics and hospitals in the 1990s.

Patients learn about ACCTs through access to a network of support organizations, usually led by former patients or family members of former patients. Those organizations provide information about a wide range of therapies. Many of the alternative therapies were founded by scientists or clinicians who had credentials and work experience that could have located them, or did locate them for some time, within the medical and scientific establishment but who because of their choice to pioneer alternatives, became controversial. Examples of researchers and clinicians who fit that category include Stanislaw Burzynski (antineoplastons), the late Lawrence Burton (immuno-augmentative therapy), Ernesto Contreras (laetrile, etc.), Joseph Gold (hydrazine sulfate), the late Virginia Livingston (autogenous bacterial vaccines), the late Harold Manner (laetrile, enzymes, and vitamin A), the late Linus Pauling (vitamin C), and the late Eli Jordon Tucker (DMSO and hematoxylon).

The controversies surrounding their research could be conceptualized in terms of the social studies of science literature as controversies within the scientific and medical communities between orthodox and unorthodox members (Hess 1997b). However, the research controversies are also connected to patients, via clinical applications, and patients and their friends have organized into a social movement. Therefore, the ACCT community is sociologically a combination of a network of researchers in a series of linked scientific controversies, a new social movement, and an incipient heterodox scientific community in which activist patients and unorthodox clinicians and researchers are working synergetically.

The relations among the scientific researchers, patients, and the leaders of patient support and referral organizations are further complicated by biographical trajectories that result in a change of roles over time. The interviews identified a pattern whereby people tended to progress from naive patient to dissatisfied user of conventional therapies, to informed consumer of ACCTs, and on to referral or support-group person. In some cases they earn advanced degrees in nutrition or a biomedical field and achieve professional positions. The trajectory is similar to those found in other biomedical social movements, such as AIDS activism (Epstein 1996).

Likewise, there are cases of clinicians who have become dissatisfied with their conventional medical practices or who have sought ACCTs in response to their own cancer or that of a family member and become journalists or writers, publicizing the cause of ACCTs. The movement back-and-forth among patients, clinicians, and researchers—mediated by journalists and patient-support organization leaders—creates a dynamic interchange that is part scientific research community and part social movement.

POSITIONS: THE POLITICS OF EVALUATION

Interviews with the researchers, clinicians, and leaders of information-providing organizations focused on the question of evaluation. The main questions in the one-to-two-hour semistructured telephone interviews were what evaluation criteria they used and which ACCTs they thought most and least promising. Over the course of the interviews I learned to distinguish various types of evaluation: (1) the patient's needs at all levels, including financial, social, spiritual, and of course biomedical; (2) referral and patient support organizations; (3) clinicians and clinical organizations (including quality of service delivery); (4) the therapies themselves; (5) a meta-level involving criteria for evaluating therapies (such as randomized, controlled trials); and (6) policies and politics of research, funding, and regulation. The themes that emerged regarding the evaluation of therapies and criteria for evaluating therapies are reviewed elsewhere (Hess 1998). This section will summarize some of the views regarding methodology.

Many of the interviewees were well aware of the politics of randomized, controlled trials for ACCTs, including documented cases of design modifications that introduced biases against ACCTs (Houston 1989; Moss 1996). A critical, sociological, and historical literature on randomized, controlled trials is now beginning to emerge (e.g., Coulter 1991; Epstein 1996; Marks 1997). One set of criticisms in our interviews focused on the economic issues that exclude small-scale clinicians from pursuing the "gold standard" of randomized, controlled trials. Likewise, the unpatentable nature of most of the ACCTs implies that pharmaceutical companies are unlikely to invest the funds required to achieve FDA approval. Since the late 1980s the FDA has approved some conventional cancer drugs without randomized, controlled trials; however, the gold standard is often demanded for nontoxic, nonpatentable therapies. As journalist Robert Houston commented in one interview (Hess 1998), the gold standard is therefore a double standard.

Other criticisms focused on the problem of how placebo controls were impossible for such therapies as the Gerson dietary program, which involves coffee enemas and a dozen glasses of juice per day. Some interviewees suggested testing clinicians and clinics as total units rather than specific therapeutic modalities, as tends to occur in conventional medicine. Others questioned the ethics of running any randomized clinical trials for late-stage cancer patients, who often request a clinical strategy of switching therapeutic modalities if the ones first attempted show no short-term benefit.

Interviewees were well aware of the hierarchy of evaluation methods and the difficulties of using retrospective outcomes analysis, case study reviews, and subclinical data as a basis for making decisions. However, notwithstanding the biopolitical situation, they often looked at all data and attempted to arrive at a holistic calculation that took into account legality, cost, ease of use, and safety. Several interviewees pointed to the outcomes analyses of Hildenbrand and colleagues (1995, 1996) as a possible model for future research and evaluation that does not compromise clinical ethics but allows for some of the rigor associated with controlled trials. In some cases, clinicians were willing to use substances that had support only at the lower rungs of the ladder of evidence if they appeared relatively safe and nontoxic, but they wanted higher levels of evidence for more toxic substances.

CONCLUSIONS

From the public understanding of science—in this case, the understanding that patients have of cancer—is still based on the transmission model. In other words, we (the medical community) know what science is, we do it, and we transmit it to you, the public and the patients, either directly (such as via the NCI website on ACCTs or the media) or indirectly (through your doctor). In its more democratic guises, the transmission model is linked to public education policies that attempt to transmit science to the "great unwashed." A less democratic guise is a policy of suppression of ACCTs and their advocates. The politics of suppression can involve FDA raids on supplements firms and clinicians, FDA refusal to approve nonpatentable and nontoxic natural substances for cancer treatment, loss of medical licenses, prosecution of holistic doctors for involvement in alleged illegal medical practices, denial of grants to researchers who go outside the mainstream, and refusal to publish research. The effects of suppression can extend to social scientists who document the suppression, under the pretense that their work is not objective or value neutral.

Notwithstanding the strong support of the transmission model in scientific and medical communities, social scientists have increasingly documented the ways in which the understandings of patients and other publics differ from those of the expert producers whose knowledges and technologies they consume (Hess 1995, ch. 5; Irwin and Wynne 1996). The alternative that emerges from research on both sides of the Atlantic is the "reconstruction model"—that is, patients (or other public groups and social movements) operate as active agents who reinterpret and question expert knowledge. However, the mere recognition that lay understandings are different from those of the experts is only half the picture. Patients not only have different understandings from those of doctors and researchers (see also Hunt, in this volume) but occasionally challenge research agendas and regulatory policies. A viable alternative to the transmission model needs to take into account not only the activity of patients and the public in their reception of expertise but also the ways in which the public shapes that expertise. It is therefore necessary to extend the reconstruction model to describe how pockets of the public coalesce into social movements and organizations that go beyond the reconstruction of expert authority. In some cases, public organizations develop their own research (such as lay epidemiology) and become involved in reshaping the research and regulatory agendas of the experts, often via alliances with unorthodox members of scientific research communities.

Consequently, a more accurate model of the relationship between the science and the public, at least for the case of ACCTs, is what I term the "public shaping of science" model. In this model, citizen groups coalesce from the public, and out of them emerge leaders who question the expertise of research establishments, produce alternative knowledge, and challenge research agendas. The process has been documented in other patient activist movements, such as repetitive-strain injury (Arksey 1994) and AIDS activism (Epstein 1996; Treichler 1991), and it is an extension of more general ways in which citizen groups affect the policy process (Peterson 1984). The case of ACCTs is distinctive, however, because of its emphasis on changing the research agenda toward the evaluation of less toxic therapies and diagnostic procedures, and because of the sophisticated quality of some of the research that has been produced.

As patients who use alternative and complementary therapies become more organized and more sophisticated about the biomedical politics of research and regulation, they have begun to have a policy impact. Such legislative reforms as the "Access to Medical Treatments" bill, which in 1999 was still pending approval in Congress, promise to give doctors and their patients the right to experiment with safe alternative therapies under conditions of informed consent. Versions of that legislation and related laws have already been passed in several state legislatures. A number of other policy reforms merit consideration and have been discussed elsewhere (Hess 1997a; Houston 1989).

Perhaps the most complicated issue of policy reform is the problem of evaluating ACCTs. As the medical community learns that the biopolitical landscape has been permanently altered, that patients and the public at large are demanding an increasing role in the shaping of scientific research agendas, the policy of suppression will be replaced by one of evaluation. In other words, whereas the transmission model leads to a policy of suppression, the model of public shaping of science suggests an alternative policy, evaluation. However, that policy cannot be embraced naively. The collective wisdom and experience of the leaders of the ACCT community note that in the cases where public support has led to clinical trials of ACCTs, trial designs have been manipulated to produce failures for ACCTs (Houston 1989; Moss 1996). Given the experience with prejudicial design alterations in trials for laetrile, vitamin C, hydrazine sulfate, and most recently antineoplastons (which Burzynski found out about during the trial, thus forcing cancellation), the interviewees were very skeptical that the major organizations associated with the cancer establishment could produce unbiased evaluations of ACCTs.

Accordingly, a policy of evaluation begins to replace a policy of suppression, there needs to be an awareness of the history of trials funded to end controversy that end up fueling it. Key figures from the ACCT community, such as Gar Hildenbrand, Robert Houston, and Ralph Moss—as well as moderate, mediating leaders such as Michael Lerner and Keith Block—need to be included in consultations over design. A number of policy checks needs to be implemented in the evaluation process. One example is the inclusion of multiple sites, including nonestablishment organizations. The design of trials might even include site as a variable, employing such major alternative institutions as Tijuana hospitals or naturopathic universities. Another policy check is to give coprincipal investigator status to the ACCT advocate of a therapy, allowing that person complete access to the test site and protocols, to ensure that protocols are not altered after being implemented.

The question of preventing and controlling cancer in North America is therefore a complicated political issue. Clearly, more research and funding needs to be devoted to prevention, and those funds should be protected from being siphoned off into such projects as trials of preventive chemotherapy. The control of cancer, however, may ultimately rest on the public control of cancer politics and research.

ACKNOWLEDGMENTS

This material is based upon work supported by the National Science Foundation under Grant No. SBR-9511543, "Public Understanding of Science." Any opinions, findings, and conclusions or recommendations expressed in this material are those of the author or interviewees and do not necessarily reflect the views of the National Science Foundation. Robert Houston made several helpful corrections for the final draft.

LITERATURE CITED

Arksey, Hilary. 1994. Expert and lay participation in the construction of medical knowledge. *Sociology of Health and Illness* 16(4):448–68.
British Medical Association. 1993. *Complementary medicine: New approaches to good medical practice*. New York: Oxford University Press.
Cassileth, Barrie, Edward Lusk, Thomas Strouse, and Brenda Brodenheimer. 1984. Contemporary unorthodox treatments in cancer medicine. *Annals of Internal Medicine* 101(1):105–112.
Coulter, Harris. 1991. *The controlled clinical trial*. Washington, DC: Project Cure, Center for Empirical Medicine.
Davis, Devra Lee, Gregg Dinse, and David Hoel. 1994. Decreasing cardiovascular disease and increasing cancer among whites in the United States from 1973 through 1987. *Journal of the American Medical Association* 271(6):431–437.
Eisenberg, David, Ronald Kessler, Cindy Foster, Frances Norlock, David Calkins, and Thomas Delbanco. 1993. Unconventional medicine in the United States. *New Eng-*

land Journal of Medicine 328(4):246-52.

Epstein, Samuel. 1992. Profiting from cancer: Vested interests and the cancer epidemic.*Ecologist* 22(5):233–240.

—. 1996. *Impure science: AIDS, activism, and the politics of knowledge.* Berkeley: University of California Press.

Furnham, A., and J. Forey. 1994. The attitudes, behaviors, and beliefs of patients of conventional versus complementary (alternative) medicine. *Journal of Clinical Psychology* 50:458–469.

Hess, David J. 1995. *Science and technology in a multicultural world.* New York: Columbia University Press.

—. 1997a. *Can bacteria cause cancer? Alternative medicine confronts big science.* New York: NYU Press.

—. 1997b. *Science studies: An advanced introduction.* New York: NYU Press.

—. 1998. *Evaluating alternative cancer therapies.* New Brunswick: Rutgers University Press.

Hildenbrand, Gar, L. Christeene Hildenbrand, Karen Bradford, and Shirley Cavin. 1995. Five-year survival rates of melanoma patients treated by diet therapy after the manner of Gerson: A retrospective review. *Alternative Therapies* 1(4): 29–37.

Hildenbrand, Gar, L. Christeene Hildenbrand, Karen Bradford, Dan E. Rogers, Charlotte Gerson Strauss, and Shirley Cavin. 1996. The role of follow-up and retrospective data analysis in alternative cancer management: The Gerson experience. *Journal of Naturopathic Medicine* 6(1):49–56.

Houston, Robert. 1989. *Repression and reform in the evaluation of alternative cancer therapies.* Washington, DC: Project Cure.

Irwin, Alan, and Brian Wynne, eds. 1996. *Misunderstanding science? The public reconstruction of science and technology.* Cambridge: Cambridge University Press.

Marks, Harry. 1997. The progress of experiment. New York: Cambridge University Press.

McGinnis, Lamar. 1991. Alternative therapies, 1990: An overview. *Cancer* 67(6 Supp.):1788–1792.

Moss, Ralph. 1995. *Questioning Chemotherapy.* Brooklyn, NY: Equinox.

—. 1996. *The cancer industry.* Brooklyn, NY: Equinox.

Parker, Sheryl, Tony Tong, Sherry Bolden, and Phyllis Wingo. 1997. Cancer statistics, 1997. *CA-A Journal for Clinicians* 47:5–27.

Peterson, James. 1984. *Citizen participation in science.* Amherst: University of Massachusetts Press.

Peterson, James, and Gerald Markle. 1979a. The laetrile controversy. In *Controversy: Politics of technical decisions,* ed. Dorothy Nelkin, 159–179. Beverly Hills, CA: Sage.

—. 1979b. Politics and science in the laetrile controversy. *Social Studies of Science* 9:139-66.

Sharma, Ursula. 1992. *Complementary medicine today: Practitioners and patients.* London and New York: Routledge.

Treichler, Paula. 1991. How to have a theory in an epidemic: The evolution of AIDS treatment activism. In *Technoculture: Cultural politics.* Vol. 3, ed. Constance Penley and Andrew Ross, 57–106. Minneapolis: University of Minnesota Press.

Wooddell, Margaret, and David Hess. 1998. *Women confront cancer.* New York: NYU Press.

Chapter 3

The Metastasis of Witchcraft: A Case Study of the Interrelationship between Traditional and Biomedical Models

Linda M. Hunt

INTRODUCTION

In the course of ethnographic research on hospital-based cancer diagnosis and treatment in southern Mexico, I found that medical staff and patient families may have very different goals on and perspectives on trying to understand and address serious illness. For physicians and medical staff, the primary task in diagnosing and treating illness is to identify biological dysfunction and then pursue a program of technical actions aimed at correcting that dysfunction. Medical staff rely primarily on a biomedical model that places biological process in the foreground (Engle 1963; Engle and Davis 1963; Kleinman 1993; Good 1994; Hunt 1994) In contrast, from the perspective of patients and their families a catastrophic illness presents a complicated set of challenges reaching well beyond the bounded universe of biology. Such an illness may introduce a major disruption into their whole lifeworld, undermining the integrity, continuity, and coherence of a sense of self and of family life (Scarry 1985; Kleinman 1988; Garro 1993, 1995; Good 1993).

Living with such an illness thus poses pressing existential problems of explanation and response. The struggles of cancer patients and their families I have interviewed to meet these challenges in addressing cancer generated complex and multifaceted illness models. These models are concerned not so much with describing and controlling biological dysfunction as with making sense of the illness in a much broader context (Hunt 1992)—striving to incorporate it into their long-term biographical reality and embark on practical actions.

I have found that while these families almost always embrace the biomedical diagnoses and treatments given them in the hospitals, they often simultaneously draw on traditional illness concepts as well. In this paper I present a rather striking example of the process by which biomedical and traditional illness concepts may be combined in their everyday application. Let me preface the discussion by emphasizing that the case I have chosen as an illustration is an extreme one. Commonly the interaction between biomedical and traditional models is a much subtler process than it will appear to be here. However, I have chosen this example because in its extremeness, it casts the syncretism of biomedical and traditional systems in high relief. I will begin with a discussion, based on interviews with the physicians and nurses involved and on review of hospital medical records, of the medical staff's perspective on the situation. I will then examine the family's perspective, as expressed in in-depth interviews with the patient's parents, conducted in their home. I conclude with an analysis of the interaction between these two perspectives.

BACKGROUND

While Mexico has an extensive national health care system, which provides access to biomedical care even in remote areas, it also has a long and elaborate tradition of the use of herbal and traditional medicines (see for example Anzures y Bolañas 1983; Ortiz de Montellano 1990). Although public clinics throughout the country offer free or low-cost biomedical care, many people, particularly in rural areas, rely on traditional remedies to treat common illnesses like stomach ache and influenza. In addition to home remedies, a variety of local folk practitioners, such as spiritual healers and *curanderos*, are also commonly used.

In my observations in southern Mexico, traditional treatment approaches are most often used in conjunction with biomedical treatments rather than instead of them. People intermix Western and non-Western health care systems in their concepts of cause, diagnosis, and treatment of illness. It has been widely demonstrated in studies throughout the world that in pluralistic health care systems, biomedical and ethnomedical practices most often complement one another rather than compete (Helman 1978; Higgins 1975; Janzen 1978; Blumhagen 1980; Cosminsky and Scrimshaw 1980; Finkler 1981; Young and Garro 1982; Cosminsky 1983; Hunt at al. 1989; Brodwin 1991). Several studies, undertaken in a variety of cultural settings, have found that people tend to move between health care systems according to their understandings of the cause of their illnesses (Brown 1963; Romanucci-Ross 1969; Nichter 1980; Young 1981; Low 1985; Garro 1988, 1990). Research in industrializing countries, such as Mexico, has shown that people often divide illnesses between those (like cancer) thought to have causes associated with modernization and those thought to have traditional causes, and that treatments are chosen accordingly (Aguirre Beltrán 1965; Rubel et al. 1984; Frazier 1981; Stebbins 1986).

In southern Mexico, as in most of the world, the biomedical model carries great cultural authority and therefore is not readily rejected. However, its relevance to the lives of patients and their families is often rather limited. In its focus on identifying and controlling salient biological processes, the biomedical model is not centrally concerned with associating the illness to broader life circumstances. At the same time, biomedical treatments often require investments of time and resources that are out of the reach of many poor patients, and therefore they may be of little use in establishing a course of practical action. In contrast, traditional ill-ness models are much more adept at accomplishing both of these tasks: explaining illness in terms salient to a specific biography, and indicating accessible therapeu-tic actions (Rubel et al. 1984; Harris 1989; Finkler 1991). Some have argued that one reason folk health care systems retain their popularity is that they serve im-plicit functions of organizing social relations and draw on a variety of culturally charged symbols in ways that the biomedical system does not (Aguirre Beltrán 1963; Adams and Rubel 1967; Finkler 1985, 1990). By combining elements from both biomedical and traditional systems, patients' families generate illness models that are able to give meaning to the illness and direct practical action as an embed-ded part of their life experiences (Hunt et al. 1990). They are thus able to begin to answer some important questions left unaddressed by the biomedical model, ques-tions like: Why us? Why now? How could this tragedy have come into our lives? What can be done to make things right again? (cf. Williams 1984; Williams and Wood 1986).

In the case presented in this paper, the family of Roberto Gomez illus-trates how traditional illness concepts address these questions. Their explanation combines biomedical and traditional concepts in a way that provides a conceptual mechanism for understanding and explaining, in socially relevant terms, the other-wise arbitrary tragedy. Their idea that illness has been caused by an object or su-pernatural force intruding into the body is a common one in Mexican folk medicine (Adams and Rubel 1967; Nader 1969; Finkler 1985). The belief that such an intru-sion can cause an illness presents a flexible and versatile idiom for locating the source of disorder within the context of an individual life history, pinpointing an attack from without that may have rendered the person sick (cf. Young 1980; Pol-lack 1988; Harris 1989; Hunt et al. 1989).

Witchcraft explanations for illness, such as the one this family used, are common throughout the world. Because such explanations ascribe illness to forces within the spiritual or social realms, they add layers of moral and social meaning to explanations of empirical cause and effect (Evans-Pritchard 1937). Attributing an illness to the action of a witch provides a causal explanation that gives moral and social meaning to illness through a language of culpability and accusation. This provides both an opportunity to measure current relationships against an ideal of social life and to make moves to adjust them.

THE CASE OF ROBERTO GÓMEZ[2]

Reviewing the transcript of an ethnographic interview conducted by my research assistant with the family of a young cancer patient in a public hospital in Chiapas, Mexico, I was impressed by the remarkable way in which the family mixed biomedical and traditional illness concepts. Throughout the interview the parents had been referring to the child's malady using terms consistent with the biomedical model, describing it as a progressive disease that required aggressive treatment and was capable of spreading and eventually killing the patient. The in-terviewer had gone on to ask a simple control question, meant to see whether the family knew the specific diagnosis: "What did the doctor tell you was the matter with your son?" I was startled at the father's response: "Witchcraft." Intrigued by this anomaly, I set out for their village, hoping to get a clearer understanding of the process by which they were combining biomedical and traditional perspectives.

The patient was Roberto Gómez, a fourteen-year-old *campesino*, or farmer. He lived with his parents and two younger brothers in a one-room hut in a village near the Guatemalan border. The nearest city, which I will call Vista Hermosa, is a market center of about 100,000 people, an hour's bus ride from Roberto's village. Roberto had been treated at the Vista Hermosa General Hospital, which serves one of the poorest and least industrialized areas of Mexico. Its catchment area includes nearly 500,000 people, about 25% of whom are ethnically Mayan and maintain many Mayan traditions (Halperin et al. 1991).

The Medical Perspective

The medical perspective on Roberto's illness may be briefly summarized. When Roberto's family brought him to the General Hospital he was very weak, barely conscious, in a great deal of pain, coughing, and had been unable to walk for several weeks. His left foot was very swollen, described by one nurse as the size of a watermelon. The foot had a raging infection that was discharging pus and was infested with maggots.

Roberto was hospitalized and remained in the hospital for the next two months. Eventually the infection was brought under control, and the presence of a large tumor in the foot was detected. A biopsy revealed an advanced case of Ewing's sarcoma, a small-cell tumor of bone that occurs most commonly in the legs and feet of children between the ages of eleven and fifteen (Falk 1988). Metastasis, or spread of the cancerous cells, to the lung was also noted. The prognosis was grave.

When the family declined to transfer Roberto to a public hospital in Mexico City for surgery and radiation treatment, Vista Hermosa doctors amputated Roberto's leg at the hip. The child suffered extreme psychological depression as a result of the amputation and showed little improvement. The family then refused to transfer the boy to another city, about five hours to the north, for palliative chemotherapy and radiation treatment, which were not available in Vista Hermosa. Instead, they opted to take the boy home, against medical advice.

From the perspective of the hospital staff, the family was ignorant and negligent in not having brought in the boy soon enough for treatment and not having kept the wound clean. The doctor said that in spite of his repeated efforts to educate the family about the diagnosis and treatment, they would not understand the information but clung instead to superstition and traditional beliefs (cf. Good et al. 1992). This stubborn ignorance was, in his view, at least partially responsible for the difficulties encountered in this case.

The Family's Perspective

Now let us consider the family's version of what happened to Roberto. I arrived in their village two months after they had left the hospital. I discovered that eight days after returning home, Roberto had died in his bed. The family was still actively mourning the loss of Roberto, openly crying and grieving through much of the interview. They told me that Roberto's illness had begun when a neighborhood boy had kicked him playing soccer. The boy's family had been feuding with Roberto's for some time over crops damaged by grazing pigs. The boy had left town five days later, and within a few weeks Roberto's foot had begun to swell and hurt.

They took him to a *huesero*, or bonesetter, who said the bone was not broken and treated the bruised area with herbal compresses. The foot continued to swell and became more and more painful. They went to another *huesero*. He also tried treating the foot with herbs for a few weeks, then told them that he thought the problem might be witchcraft.

They consulted a medical doctor in a small government clinic in a nearby village. He told them it was "too late," that he could not help them. He said they needed to take Roberto to the big public hospital in Mexico City. This seemed impossible to the family: Mexico City was very far away. They had never been there but had heard many stories that it was very expensive to get there and very difficult and dangerous to stay there once you arrived. They could not imagine how they might travel to Mexico City with a sick child. In their view, this doctor had not offered them any realistic solutions, had not helped them at all. They continued seeking a solution among the traditional practitioners in their community.

Combining the opinions of various curers and family members, Roberto's family came to believe that a supernatural *coral*, or snake, had been sent by the neighbor family to harm Roberto. It had intruded into his body when he was kicked by their son. Several times over the ensuing months, Roberto had awakened crying in the night, dreaming that the *coral* had come to eat from his foot. Once his mother had seen it slither out the doorway when she came into the room where Roberto was sleeping.

Over the next few months they took Roberto to several spiritists and *curanderos* in an attempt to cure him of the witchcraft. They spent a great deal of money in the endeavor. The illness only continued to worsen. The frustrated family did not know what else to try. One day a sister-in-law came to visit them and found Roberto very ill with a raging fever, a horribly swollen foot, and a great deal of pain. She insisted that they take the boy immediately to the Vista Hermosa Hospital, which was several hours away by bus.

At the hospital, the doctors unbandaged the wound and found that it was infested with *gusanos*, worms. The family had just cleaned the wound that morning, so they knew the *gusanos* could not be there because it was dirty. It was clear to them that they were from the *coral's* multiplying in the boy's body.

When the doctors amputated the leg, they showed the family what they had found inside: Roberto's father described it as "lumps of meat." After the amputation, Roberto was worse than ever. He was unable to walk, developed a bad cough, and was extremely sad and confused about the loss of his leg. The doctors said the disease was spreading through his body and had begun to damage the lungs. The father explained to me that this was due to the *gusanos* traveling through the bones, spreading the illness to the lungs and other parts of the body.

They were told that there was no cure but that there was a treatment in another city that could slow the process, perhaps prolong Roberto's life a few months. Over the past year the family had already sold all of their land and live-stock to pay for the various treatments. They were destitute. Wasn't this just one more treatment that wasn't going to work? They decided to take Roberto home instead.

Roberto lived eight more days, coughing and crying with pain. When he died it was an end to many long months of suffering. Although the neighbor family refused to admit that they had sent the *coral*, Roberto's family remained convinced that they were behind the illness. The tangible evidence had clearly supported this notion: How could the "lumps of meat" and the *gusanos* have gotten into his foot except by witchcraft? The *coral* had been seen in the doorway and in dreams. The neighbor's son had disappeared after he had done the deed. Who else but that family would have had a motive to send such misery to Roberto's family?

DISCUSSION

In the biomedical version of what happened to Roberto, the meaningful events were hidden at the cellular level: cancerous cells were reproducing and mi-grating through the body. The recommended actions focused on applying sophisti-cated technologies in order to destroy those cells: technologies that were virtually inaccessible to the family (cf. Hunt 1995). Such an explanation had little salience for them. It did not connect the illness in any meaningful way to their life experi-ence, nor did it provide a viable course of action. The family encountered the ill-ness not as the manifestation of obscure biological events but as a profoundly em-bedded part of their unfolding life experience. To give the illness meaning and embark on a workable plan of action in this context, the family generated a very different kind of illness explanation.

In their view, the illness had begun with the *golpe*, or blow, when Roberto was kicked by the neighbor boy.[3] From the biomedical perspective, this event was incidental, unimportant to the process of cellular dysfunction. For the family, how-ever, the *golpe* was key. It was an identifiable moment in which there was a breach of the boundaries between Roberto and exterior forces. This was a moment in which the child could be bewitched: by means of the *golpe* the *coral* could intrude into his body. In contrast, the biomedical model did not address the question of how the errant cells may have entered the child's leg.

By drawing on traditional beliefs about witchcraft and *golpes*, the family was able to answer two pressing question about the illness that were not considered by the biomedical model: How did the illness begin? Who had the moral responsi-bility for the invasion? From the perspective of the medical staff, the several months spent in consultations with *hueseros*, spiritists, and *curanderos* were simply wasted time. For the family, however, these treatments made much more practical sense than going to the medical doctor. When they had first consulted with a physician they had been told it was "too late" to be treated by him and that they needed to go to Mexico City: an utterly impossible undertaking from their point of view. Embracing this model would have meant giving up hope. Instead they concentrated on the witchcraft model, which offered both a tangible explanation and feasible action.

When finally the family came in desperation to the hospital, the medical staff interpreted the *gusanos*, or maggots, in the wound as evidence of poor hygiene and of negligence. The family, rather than accept the moral responsibility for this late-developing event, readily fit it into their ongoing explanation: the *gusanos* were empirical evidence of the presence of the *coral*, or snake. When the child developed symptoms of lung disease, the biomedical model attributed it to metastatic spread of cancerous cells, which required chemotherapy and radiation: treatments to which the family felt they had no access. Again, thinking in terms of cellular process had no meaning for the family. So, while they accepted the idea that the disease was indeed spreading, they integrated that idea with their own concepts of the illness, concluding that the *gusanos* had traveled through the body and attacked the lungs. The resulting combined model envisions a hybrid construct: a metastasis of witchcraft. Thus the biomedical model, as interpreted by this family, was used to underwrite and confirm their traditional beliefs.

Given that medical treatment was no more effective in curing the child than the traditional treatments had been, the family's incorporation of traditional and biomedical explanations seems logical. By embracing the biomedical model the family invoked the technical authority of modern medicine. However, because they had very limited access to the recommended treatments, the model in effect shut them out. It was therefore of limited practical relevance for them. The witchcraft model, on the other hand, assigned individual agency to the enemy family. It thereby connected the catastrophic illness in a meaningful way to the family's broader life story. At the same time it indicated a set of accessible actions that were socially and morally relevant (cf. Das 1995).

CONCLUSION

Although no other patients in my research evoked witchcraft as a specific cause of cancer, this case clearly illustrates the process of combining biomedical and traditional medical systems as I have consistently observed it in my work with Mexican cancer patients. The medical version of what is happening to a patient focuses on biological process. It reduces events to terms salient to the biomedical model (Eisenberg and Kleinman 1980; Hahn and Gaines 1985; Lock and Gordon 1988) and recommends treatments that are often not readily accessible to patients. In contrast, patient families' models are often quite broad in focus. They identify adverse situations from their life circumstances as both cause and consequence of the illness (cf. Horton 1970; Harris 1989; Pandolfi 1990; Hunt in press), and are thereby able to initiate therapeutic actions that are readily available. Thus, traditional models generate explanations and actions that are much more salient in the context of the everyday lifeworld than are those generated by the biomedical model.

Still, in spite of its much narrower focus, the biomedical model does carry great social authority and technical promise. Even though families may lack access to recommended treatments, the medical explanation is seldom rejected; instead, it is often interwoven with more morally and practically relevant traditional explanations. Patient family explanations may combine the authoritative meaning generated in the biomedical model with the specific and accessible meanings found in traditional models. Thus, the social authority of biomedical explanations may be used to underwrite and confirm concepts generated by traditional models. Biomedical and traditional models are not perceived by patient families to be contradictory but rather as compatible elements of an evolving illness understanding. By drawing on both traditional and biomedical systems, families are able to address both the pressing existential question of how things could go so wrong and the practical question of what can be done to make things right again.

ACKNOWLEDGMENTS

This paper is based upon research supported in part by the following grants: National Science Foundation #BNS 8916157; Wenner-Gren #Gr.5183; Fundación México en Harvard Research Grant; and a University of North Carolina at Charlotte Faculty Research Grant. Any opinions, findings, conclusions, or recommendations expressed in this paper are mine and do not necessarily reflect the views of these foundations. I wish to thank Imelda Martinez for her invaluable help in interviewing and transcribing. I also wish to express my gratitude for the cooperation and support of the Centro de Investigaciones de Salud de Comitán, Chiapas, México, and to the patients and physicians whose cooperation made this research possible.

NOTES

1. Originally published in 1993. *Collegium Antropologicum* 17(2):249–256. Reprinted by permission of the Institute for Anthropological Research.
2. All proper names are pseudonyms.
3. Studies have found that *golpes*, or blows, are commonly mentioned by Mexicans and Mexican Americans as a cause of cancer (Hunt 1992; Chavez et al. 1995).

LITERATURE CITED

Adams, R., and A. Rubel. 1967. Sickness and social relations. In *Handbook of Middle American Indians*, vol. 6, ed. R. Wauchope, 333–356. Austin: University of Texas Press.
Aguirre Beltrán, Gonzales. 1963. *Medicina y magia: El proceso de aculturación en la*

Estructura Colonial. México, DF: Instituto Naciónal Indigenista.

—. 1965. *Los programas de salud en la situación intracultural*. México, DF: Instituto Nacional Indigenista.

Anzures y Bolañas, María del Carmen. 1977. La medicina tradicional ¿Factor de cambio en la medicina oficial de México? *Los Procesos de Cambio* 15(1):305–312.

Blumhagen, Dan. 1980. Hypertension: A folk illness with a medical name. *Culture, Medicine and Psychiatry* 4:197–227.

Brodwin, Paul. 1991. Political contests and moral claims: Religious pluralism and healing in a Haitian village. Ph.D. dissertation, Harvard University.

Brown, Jack. 1963. Some changes in Mexican village curing practices induced by western medicine. *America Indigena* 23(2):93–120.

Chavez, L., A. Hubbell, J. McMullin, R. Shiraz, I. Mishra, and R. Valdez. 1995. Structure and meaning in models of breast and cervical cancer risk factors: A comparison of perceptions among Latinas, Anglo women, and physicians. *Medical Anthropology* 9(1):40–74.

Cosminsky, Sheila and Mary Scrimshaw. 1980. Medical pluralism on a Guatemala plantation. *Social Science and Medicine* 14B:267–278.

Cosminsky, Sheila. 1983. Medical pluralism in Mesoamerica. In *Heritage of conquest: Thirty years later,* ed. C. Kendall et al., 159–173. Albuquerque: University of New Mexico Press.

Das, V. 1995. *Critical events: Anthropological perspectives on contemporary India*. Delhi: Oxford University Press.

Eisenberg, L., and A. Kleinman eds. 1980. *The relevance of social science for medicine*. Dordrecht: D. Reidel.

Engle, R. 1963. Medical diagnosis: Past, present and future—II. Philosophical foundations and historical developments of our concepts of health, disease and diagnosis. *Archives Internal Medicine* 112:520–529.

Engle, R. J., and B. J. Davis. 1963. Medical diagnosis: Past, present and future—I. Present concepts on the meaning and limitations of medical diagnosis. *Archives Internal Medicine* 112:512–519.

Evans-Pritchard, E. E. 1937. *Witchcraft, oracles and magic among the Azande*. Oxford: Clarendon.

Falk, P. 1988. Cancers in childhood. In *Manual of Clinical Oncology*, ed. D. Casciato and B. Lowitz, 272-281. Boston: Little Brown.

Finkler, K. 1981. A comparative study of health seekers: Or, why do some people go to the doctor rather than to a spiritualist healer. *Medical Anthropology* 5(4):383–424.

—. 1985. *Spiritualist healers in Mexico: Successes and failures of alternative therapeutics*. New York: Praeger.

—. 1991. *Physicians at work, patients in pain: Biomedical practice and patient response in Mexico*. Boulder, CO: Westview Press.

Frazier, Robert. 1981. Progress in the delivery of health care in Mexico. *Pediatrics* 67(1):155–157.

Garro, Linda C. 1988. Continuity and change: Medical knowledge and the interpretation of illness in a Canadian Ojibwa community. Paper presented at the 12th International Congress of Anthropological and Ethnological Sciences, Zagreb, Yugoslavia.

—. 1990. Culture, pain and cancer. *Journal of Palliative Care* 6(3):34–44.

—. 1993. Chronic illness and the construction of narratives. In *Pain as human experience: Anthropological studies in American culture*, eds. M. J .D. Good et al., 100–137. Los Angeles: University of California Press.

—. 1995. Individual or societal responsibility? Explanations of diabetes in an Anishinaabe

(Ojibway) community. *Social Science and Medicine* 40(1):37–46. Good, Byron. 1993. A body in pain: The making of a world of chronic pain. In *Pain as human experience: Anthropological studies in American culture*, ed. M. J. D. Good et al., 29-48. Los Angeles: University of California Press.

—. 1994. *Medicine, rationality and experience: An anthropological perspective.* Cambridge: Cambridge University Press.

Good, M. D., L. M. Hunt, T. Munakata, and Y. Kobayash. 1992. A comparative analysis of the culture of biomedicine: Disclosure and consequences for treatment in the practice of oncology. In *Health and health care in developing societies: Sociological perspectives*, ed. P. Conrad and E. Gallagher, 18–210. Philadelphia: Temple University Press.

Hahn, Robert, and Atwood Gaines, eds. 1985. *Physicians of western medicine: Anthropological approaches to theory and practice.* Dordrecht: D. Reidel.

Halperin, D., P. Farías, and R. Tinoco. 1991. *Comitan Center for Health Research: studies of Mexico's southern border.* First Report. Comitan, Chiapas: Comitan General Hospital.

Harris, G. 1989. Mechanism and morality in patients' views of illness and injury. *Medical Anthropology Quarterly* 3(1):3.

Helman, Cecil. 1978. "Feed a cold, starve a fever"—folk models of infection in an English suburban community, and their relation to medical treatment. *Culture, Medicine and Psychiatry* 2:107–137.

Higgins, Cheleen. 1975. Integrative aspects of folk and western medicine among urban poor of Oaxaca. *Anthropology Quarterly* 48(1): 31–37.

Horton, R. 1970. African traditional thought and western science. In *Rationality*, ed. B. Wilson, 131–171. New York: Harper and Row.

Hunt, Linda M. 1992. Living with cancer in Oaxaca, Mexico: Patient and physician perspectives in cultural context. Ph.D. dissertation, Harvard University.

—. 1994. Practicing oncology in provincial Mexico: A narrative analysis. *Social Science and Medicine* 38(6):843.

—. 1995. Inequalities in the Mexican national health care system: Problems in managing cancer in southern Mexico. In *Society, health and disease: Transcultural perspectives*, ed. J. Subedi and E. Gallagher, 130–147. Upper Saddle River, NJ: Prentice-Hall.

—. In press. Strategic suffering: Illness narratives as social empowerment among Mexican cancer patients. In *Narrative and the cultural construction of illness and healing*, ed. C. Mattingly and L. Garro. Berkeley: University of California Press.

Hunt, L. M., Browner, C. H., and B. Jordan. 1990. Hypoglycemia: Portrait of an illness construct in everyday use. *Medical Anthropology Quarterly* 4(2):191–210.

Hunt, L. M., B. Jordan, and S. Irwin. 1989. Views of what's wrong: Diagnosis and patients' concepts of illness. *Social Science and Medicine* 28(9):945–956.

Janzen, John. 1978. *The quest for therapy: Medical pluralism in lower Zaire.* Berkeley: University of California Press.

Kleinman, Arthur. 1988. *The illness narratives: Suffering, healing and the human condition.* New York: Basic Books.

—. 1993. What is specific to western medicine. In *Companion encyclopedia of the history of medicine*, ed. W. Bynum and R. Porter, 15–23. London: Routledge and Kegan Paul.

Lock, Margaret, and Deborah Gordon eds. 1988. *Biomedicine examined.* Kluwer Academic Publishers: Dordrecht.

Low, Setha. 1985. *Culture, politics and medicine in Costa Rica: An anthropological study of medical change.* Bedford Hills, NY: Redgrave.

Nader, Laura. 1969. The Zapotec of Oaxaca. In *Handbook of Middle American Indians,* vol. 7, *Ethnology,* Part I, ed. R. Wauchope, 329–359. Austin: University of Texas Press.

Nichter, Mark. 1980. The layperson's perception of medicine as perspective into the utilization of multiple therapy systems in the Indian context. *Social Science and Medicine* 14B:225–233.

Ortiz de Montellano, Bernard. 1990. *Aztec medicine, health and nutrition.* New Brunswick, NJ: Rutgers University Press.

Pandolfi, M. 1990. Boundaries inside the body: Women's suffering in southern peasant Italy. *Culture, Medicine and Psychiatry* 14(2):255–273.

Pollock, K. 1988. On the nature of social stress: Production of a modern mythology. *Social Science and Medicine* 26(3):381.

Romanucci-Ross, Lola. 1969. The hierarchy of resort in curative practices: The Admiralty Islands, Melanesia. *Journal of Health and Social Behavior* 10:201–209.

Rubel, A., C. O'Nell, and R. Collado-Ardon. 1984. *Susto: A folk illness.* Berkeley: University of California Press.

Scarry, E. 1985. *The body in pain: The making and unmaking of the world.* New York: University Press.

Stebbins, K. R. 1986. Politics, economics and health services in rural Oaxaca. *Human Organization* 45(2):112–119.

Williams, G. 1984. The genesis of chronic illness: Narrative re-construction. *Sociology of Health and Illness* 6:175.

Williams, G., and P. Wood. 1986 Patients and their illnesses. *Lancet* 20/27:1435–1437.

Young, Allan. 1980. The discourse on stress and the reproduction of conventional knowledge. *Social Science and Medicine* 14B:133–146.

Young, James. 1981. *Medical choice in a Mexican village.* New Brunswick, NJ: Rutgers University Press.

Young, James, and Linda Garro. 1982. Variations in the choice of treatment in two Mexican communities. *Social Science and Medicine* 16:1453–1465.

Chapter 4

African-American Women and Breast Cancer: Failures of Biomedicine?

Rhonda J. Moore

INTRODUCTION

African Americans suffer from a significant variety of chronic illnesses and diseases (Lorde 1980, 1984; Krieger and Sidney 1996; Centers for Disease Control 1998; Wingo et al. 1998). Gender, class, and racial differences mediate an individual's experiences of health and the realities of illness and survival. For example, breast cancer incidence, mortality, and survival vary widely among women of different racial and ethnic backgrounds. The overall age-adjusted cancer mortality rate has been increasing in the United States for as long as such statistics have been kept; this trend only recently reversed, and a general decline in cancer mortality began to be noted in 1991. One important consequence of this general decline in mortality is Western biomedicine's recent proclamation and definition of cancer as an increasingly *curable and survivable disease* (Gregg et al. 1994, 524; Wingo et al. 1998). This definition persists despite the fact that the survival and cure of breast cancer is a fairly scarce resource, one that is unevenly distributed across cancer patients.

Following Kleinman, I define biomedicine in terms of its "emphasis on the scientific paradigm that is at the core of the medical profession's knowledge generating and training system" (1995, 26). In no arena has biomedicine gained such primacy over the production of these "objective, medical knowledges and practices" as it has in breast cancer research. A recent "Cancer Report Card" (CRC) jointly issued by the National Cancer Institute (NCI), the American Cancer Society (ACS), and the Centers for Disease Control and Prevention (CDCP), has also given a stamp of approval, affirming the curing powers of Western biomedicine and noting that new cases of all types of cancer have dropped for men and women of every race, with one notable exception: African-American men, due in part to the sharp rise in recently diagnosed prostate cancer cases (Wingo et al. 1998).

Overall breast cancer incidence has leveled off, and the breast cancer death rate is declining in non-Hispanic white and Hispanic women (Wingo et al. 1998). These statistics, released in March 1998, reflect observations from 1973 to 1995, the latest year for which national data is available. The 1996 numbers showed the first decline since the 1950s. These differences have been generally attributed to a combination of earlier detection, through more widespread use of screening mammography, and more effective systemic treatment, particularly at the earliest stages of disease (Wingo et al. 1998).

While the decline in mortality has been noted in white and Hispanic women, these annual rates increased for African-American women. The African-American women's higher rate did not budge from 27.5 per 100,000 (Centers for Disease Control 1998). While the mortality rates of white women with breast cancer are actually decreasing, amongst African-American women these numbers are actually increasing (Lorde 1980, 1984; American Cancer Society 1997; Wojcik et al. 1998; Centers for Disease Control 1998). African Americans receive less and worse health care than whites, meaning that they are sicker than whites and typically die at about age seventy, six or seven years earlier than whites (Centers for Disease Control 1998). Breast cancer is a disease that disproportionately affects African-American women, in terms of decreased survival.

My purpose here is not to reify racial determinism as biological or genetic determinism. Instead, I want to emphasize the historical, cultural, and political contexts that inform some of these experiences of illness and decreased survival from breast cancer in African-American women. The dilemma posed by the persistence of decreased survival in African-American women led me to ask certain questions: Are African-American breast cancer survivors failures of biomedicine? Are they perceived by the biomedical community, and by physicians in particular, as a population of women who are just going to die anyway? This seems to be the case, since most of the clinical literature suggests one or more of the following themes: (1) African-American women do not comply adequately with clinical treatment regimens; (2) they present themselves at later stages of disease; (3) they simply have more aggressive tumors; and by default, (4) they have fewer prognostic factors that would enhance their survival from this disease.

In what ways do these perceptions of death, which are constantly mediated by worst-case scenarios, late presentation of disease, and statistics, influence the physician-patient interactions so as possibly to affect the treatment of these women? Perhaps more importantly, how do these encounters look, in the eyes of these survivors? In other words, what are the messages that these women are receiving about their cancers, about their selves, about their bodies, and of course, about survival?

African-American women have a unique relationship to breast cancer, since they embody three social statuses that have been historically discriminated against and devalued: being African American, being female, and having cancer. Though the link between perceived discrimination, health, and disease has often been muted in the clinical literatures, these experiences have clinical effects (Gregg and Curry 1994).

An African-American breast cancer survivor's perceptions of self, body, and emotion are bombarded with realities that articulate the diseased aspects of the body. These assaults are threatening to a racial and gendered self, one that has already been socially, medically, and historically devalued. As such, being African American, being female, and having cancer cannot be limited only to a symbolic field and to symbolic processes. The signs used for constructing racial, gender, or cancer survivors in groupings have potentially far-reaching consequences beyond these symbolic forms. All are disempowering experiences that effect the experience of health, illness, and in this case, disease.

Persistent discrimination has the power to alienate the person (in this case African-American breast cancer survivors) from their own self-image, such that it metaphorically breaks the human body (Fanon 1968). Of course, this does not mean that women do not resist the almost immobilizing, persistent discrimination, as perceived within the context of the powerful, "rationalistic" paradigm of biomedicine, nor does it mean that they necessarily forgive these disempowering and overwhelming discourses of biomedicine and of life. What it does mean is that we need to broaden our concept of "survival from cancer." This understanding begins by realizing that the persistence of "differential mortality from breast cancer in African-American women" is more than just a symbolic death sentence, since cancer is linked with culturally informed conceptions of illness, disease course, race, history, and gender. What follows in this chapter is an examination of the experiences of perceived discrimination in the physician-patient interaction, and of the cultural effects of these perceptions on the experiences in a population of underserved African-American breast cancer survivors who were participants in a psychosocial-oncology study.

METHODS

The research on which this article was based was part of a larger qualitative and quantitative study that investigated the broad cultural dimensions in the experience of breast cancer, as well as individual survivors' personal experiences with the disease. This research was carried out in the San Francisco Bay area and in Houston, Texas, from 1996 to 1998. The participant criteria for the study were as follows: female, between twenty-seven and eighty-five years of age, and a breast cancer survivor. Part of this research was conducted through interviews with participants of the Sisters Network Support Group™ in Houston, a national African–American breast cancer survivor support organization. Other individuals were recruited through word of mouth, from the Internet, and through the Community Breast Health Project in Palo Alto, California. Our study population consisted of a small cohort of twenty-eight African-American breast cancer survivors from Houston and the San Francisco Bay area and twenty-five white women from the San Francisco Bay area. This article is based on the data collected from the African-American breast cancer survivors. The interviewer collected at the initial meeting demographic data on each participant's race/ethnicity, income, date of diagnosis, treatment regimen, and date of birth. Informed consent was obtained from each study participant at this point.

One means of achieving a greater understanding of culturally diverse populations is the use of qualitative and ethnographic methods. Using qualitative methods, such as in-depth interviews and focus groups, I investigated the meanings of social support for African-American breast cancer survivors within the cultural context of perceived discrimination. The study also assessed the effects of life stress and how their perceived deletions from breast cancer's cultural discourse of "life" affected relationships. There are few ethnographic explorations of the relationships between public discourses about cancer and the reception and effects of these discourses on the cancer behaviors of underserved and minority women. Encounters with these discourses can have real impact on the health seeking behaviors of women in these populations (Ashing-Giwa et al. 1997; Moore 1998). Ethnographic and qualitative methodologies can help researchers to extract important information about the similarities and differences in the health practitioner-patient relationship in both standard and underserved clinical cancer populations.

The interviews, which were tape recorded and transcribed, were semistructured and open-ended, allowing the subjects to express the wide range of their thoughts and feelings on the topics addressed. Subjects spoke about finding out that they had breast cancer, its effects on their social and family lives, social support, their medical and family histories, and their perceptions of how they were treated by health professionals. Qualitative research enabled me to obtain a better grasp of a woman's understandings of her illness experience, the ways in which her perceptions of her world influence how she feels about her self and her cancer, how she copes, and the ways she seeks social support. By answering open-ended questions, the subjects showed that knowledge about breast cancer and trust in their relations with their physicians is related to beliefs in the efficacy of the treatments as well as to treatment decisions. These interviews took approximately three hours.

THE NARRATIVES

While Western biomedicine has defined cancer as an increasingly curable and survivable disease, it has tended to ignore the cultural and psychological effects of these experiences in underserved cancer patients. Consequently, it has also narrated a public past that links the discovery of cancer of the breast in underserved women with a potential death sentence. How does it feel to get a symbolic death sentence? How does it feel to be narrated out of life?

An important point must be made here. Much of the literature discusses the subjectivity of African-American patients that they are either unaware, fatalistic, or superstitious; they are deemed to place an overwhelming emphasis on either "faith in folk models of illness" or in healing by God. At other times, these women are characterized as victims who lack official medical knowledge of their bodies, who are noncompliant, difficult, or hard to reach. These arguments are informed by a cultural, symbolic, and political context that has served inadvertently to *disconnect* medical practitioners from understanding these particular patients' cultural and emotional worlds (Lerman et al. 1993a, 1993b; Gregg et al. 1994). If patients are not asked what they feel, what they think, what this illness means in the context of their lives, or what matters in the their lives, such misconceptions will persist.

The African-American survivors who chose to participate in this study were very aware that the *statistics* were against them, but no one had taken the time to ask them how they felt about these issues. In this study, I wanted to understand their interpretations of "research findings" in light of their personal and clinical experiences with the disease.

My goal in these interviews was to ascertain what African-American women thought were some of the reasons for their decreased survival from breast cancer. In this regard, I attempted to ascertain the levels of biomedical knowledge that these patients had received from doctors and other health care professionals. I also tried to learn what the patients had researched on their own in order to begin to become "advocates for their care." I listened for key biomedical terminology, such as "chemotherapy," "radiation," and "lumpectomy." Then—retrospectively, since most of the interviewees had already been diagnosed and had received treatment— I asked these women what these terms meant in light of their experiences. For example, I asked them if they had heard about these terms prior to their specific diagnosis, in order to obtain a sense of the context of their medical knowledge. From these questions I asked how this biomedical knowledge fit into, or was excluded from, their lives prior, during, and after their initial encounters with cancer, cancer treatments, and survival from breast cancer.

AFRICAN-AMERICAN WOMEN AND STRESS: THE ROLE OF THE HEART

Many of the African-American breast cancer survivors with whom I spoke had a narrative about why they got breast cancer. The search for meaning after crisis and the experience of uncertainty is characteristic of the impact of cancer on these women's lives. The threat of death, as mediated by one's encounter with cancer, strikes at the heart, at the self, and at one's relationship with significant others. It presents a challenge for everyday functioning and everyday reality. In their search for meaning, many attributed their initial encounter with the disease to an intense series of psychological and emotionally stressful upheavals and losses in their lives. One common thread in the narratives explored the effects of loss, though the explication of the loss took two overlapping forms: external and internal responses to stress.

In many of these situations, loss was initially determined to be external to the self: loss of livelihood, divorce, the death of a spouse, a son's murder, or a daughter's drug use. Other women also spoke about a loss that affected an internal state of being, the heart. This internal organ existed in a broken state from a lack of love, respect, and social support. The perception of heartbreak as a central component of their past and present experiences of loss as human beings, as racial and gendered subjects, and as cancer survivors, coexisted with feelings of being taken for granted. Recurrent heartbreak and the state of being repeatedly taken for granted became metaphors for states of bodily disease that affected a woman's lived emotional and psychological experiences.

The relevance of loss and its relationship to heartbreak in African-American women was not immediately apparent. One day, a woman, Cheryl, who is Stage I and age forty-six, suggested that when I asked women why they thought that they got breast cancer, I also ask them how their hearts felt and how a broken heart caused breast cancer. She claimed:

And don't forget to ask Black women if they are broken hearted and why they are broken hearted. If you ask them why they got cancer don't forget to ask them that, that is why they got cancer, they were taken for granted by men, by family, by everyone, which leads to a broken heart, and it does not just happen once, it is a series, and since she is taken for granted she has no time to heal herself or to take time to release the stress. Yeah, you ask them why they got breast cancer [Cheryl, June 1997].

Michelle Rosaldo has argued that the heart is both a material as well as symbolic organ. The heart unites thought and feeling, inner spiritual realities, and social worlds in terms of the cultural meanings of emotions such as anger, jealousy, mistrust, and desirable consequences (Rosaldo 1980, 36). The meanings attributed to the loss that accompany broken-heartedness, breast cancer, and the feelings of being taken for granted were described in and through talk about the exploitation of African-American women's hearts, and the heart's emotional, psychic, and physiological reactions to these feelings. Loss and heartbreak coexist. They permeate the experience of living as an African-American woman, as an African-American woman with children, and then later as an African-American woman with breast cancer. This is not to say that the women did not experience joy and happiness; rather, a woman's relationship to joy and happiness, at least retrospectively, was always seen to have existed as part of tension, mediated by class and race, as loss and heartbreak invariably reared their ugly heads. I came to view pain and experience of loss in terms of how a woman's heart had been broken, how she coped with disappointment, how life had pained her, and how she had healed. Attention to the heart in this regard, and to the social, economic, political, and spiritual embodiment of these experiences by the survivor, in terms of its physiological, cultural, and psychosocial effects, can illuminate our cross-cultural understandings of health and disease progression (Rosaldo 1980, 36; Rosaldo 1993).

African-American women invariably occupy a unique role in families. In many families they are often the sole social, emotional, and economic support to children and elderly parents. To some degree they also represent the heart of families and the conduit to love and support for children. In this study, African-American women tended to get the disease younger than did the white women. African-American women were more likely to have a lower income, less likely to be married, and likely to have more children than their white female counterparts.

The status of African-American women in families as heads of households and as primary guardians has been much maligned by social theorists in the realm of social theory, and also by politicians. For example, in the mid 1960s, Daniel Moynihan authored *The Negro Family: The Case for National Action*. In this report he attributed the rise of drug abuse and out-of-wedlock births in African-American female-headed households to the matriarchal nature of the African-American family. These families, and the women who headed them, were seen as mothers of pathology, transmitters of degraded and unevolved social values, and as burdens on the welfare state. Consequently, African-American families were (and to some extent still are) labeled as inferior to white middle class families (Moynihan 1965; Gutman 1976; Davis 1994).

These earlier studies failed (as do many recent ones) to explore the social, economic, and political dynamics of what actually occurs in African-American families (Staples 1993). A variety of factors explain the overabundance of African-American female-headed households. Two examples come to mind: the increasing numbers of African-American men in prisons, and the high mortality rate of African-American men in inner cities (King 1993; Taylor-Gibbs et al.1988). Obviously, in these situations, African-American women receive from these male counterparts less economic and emotional support for their life situations. In this regard, a lack of support from society as well as from significant others invariably leads to increased life stress. Life stress has been shown to compound other stressors, including illness and disease (Sapolsky 1994; Chapman et al. 1997). There is also evidence that stress plays a role in the development and recurrence of cancer. Stress, including social stress, causes tumors to grow faster in laboratory rats and renders the rats' bodies less capable of rejecting an implanted tumor (Sapolsky 1994, 146–147). In the case of African-American women, the articulation of racial, class, and gender discrimination, as experienced by the survivor, adds many dimensions to already stressful experiences having health effects.

Stress may be exacerbated if one is deleted from the discourse of survivorship. Lauren, another office clerk, was forty-one when she found her lump in a breast self-exam. I met Lauren in Houston. I asked her if she would mind speaking with me about breast cancer; she stopped me and said, "I will tell you all about my experiences with breast cancer, my surgeries and how I feel about myself." She was very direct. We met two days later. Over coffee, at her house, she told me that she was diagnosed with two cancers: intraductal carcinoma of the breast and inflammatory breast cancer. Both were in the same breast, her right one. She says that her breast had been hot and swollen. She had felt that something was wrong, so she had told her primary care physician about it. The hot and swollen feeling persisted, and she found a lump. She received her health services at a small overburdened community clinic and she was to wait five weeks for an appointment. She told me about finding the lump:

I remember standing in the shower and doing my breast exam. It was weird and then I felt it. At first I was afraid of the lump. I checked and checked again and then I realized that I was "too young" to have breast cancer. I thought that breast cancer did not happen to women who were just over forty. Then I decided to call my doctor. I told him how I had found my lump. The doctor assured me, saying that "it was probably benign. I had nothing to worry about but that I could come in and make an appointment." So I made an appointment to see him. I demanded that he biopsy the lump. I just wanted to know if it was cancer. I had the biopsy, and then later found out that the lump was malignant and that it was cancer. I should have known! Everyone in my family has cancer, not breast cancer, but cancer. I guess nothing prepares you for cancer. Even if your family gets it, it isn't your body 'til that happens.

I found out one was intraductal carcinoma of the breast and I had another cancer in the same breast [pause] inflammatory breast cancer. I wasn't told anything else by my doctor. He told me that I had inflammatory breast cancer and that I had the other cancer. The next part of it was so confusing. I saw a surgeon and a plastic surgeon. I remember that I was confused and overwhelmed. They suggested that I have a mastectomy. I told them, "I did not care how long the operation took, I just wanted to wake up with a breast." I was on that table for eleven hours but when I woke up I had a breast [Lauren, June 1997].

Survival in all instances of cancer is linked to early detection and treatment, especially in the case of fast-growing and aggressive cancers (Murphy 1997). Inflammatory breast cancer is quite rare, but it is one of the most aggressive and fast growing breast cancers. Even without lymph node involvement, a patient's staging of disease would be either Stage IIIb or Stage IV (Murphy et al. 1997).

Lauren also showed me her scars and her newly reconstructed breast. She had a tram-flap and a reconstruction. She states:

I had a tummy tuck and a breast all in one day [laughs, then falls silent and starts to cry]. They just sent me home to die. I know they wrote me off now. Inflammatory is so aggressive. One doctor [the second opinion] even told me that to take chemo might hurt me and not help me at all. I know if I had been a white girl this wouldn't have happened, they would have talked to me more. I just know it [Lauren, June 1997].

African-American women with breast cancer have three statuses that have been negatively evaluated by the society: being African-American, being female, and having cancer. There is some relationship between low rank in a particular community and increased stress levels (Sapolsky 1994; Fox et al. 1997). In a study of baboons in the Serengeti, Sapolsky found that there is an association between the social rank of the individual and the ways in which her/his body responds to stress. (Sapolsky 1994, 264). Higher-ranking individuals within a social, political, or historical milieu receive more social support. Low-ranking individuals probably perceive that they receive less support. Moreover, while low-ranking individuals probably need more support, they are less likely to receive as many tangible resources from a system (Sapolsky 1994; Fox et al. 1997). More research needs to be done to examine this link between chronic illness, social support, immune function, rank, cultural difference, and stress.

SOCIAL SUPPORT

Clinical and experiential studies have suggested that social support increases the cancer survivor's quality of life. Research from the field of psychosocial oncology has indicated the crucial role of social support in the length of survival of cancer patients and overall quality of life (Greer 1991; Fawzy 1994, 1995; Spiegel 1993). Social isolation increases mortality risk from cancer (Fawzy 1994, 1995; Spiegel 1993; Spiegel et al. 1996). Fawzy et al., in a short-term, structured, six-week psychiatric intervention for individuals with malignant melanoma, learned that treatment subjects had decreased anxiety and depression as well as higher levels of Natural Killer Cell activity. This status predicted lower rates of recurrence and significantly better survival than controls at five–six year follow-ups (Fawzy 1993, 1994; Murphy et al. 1997). One breast cancer study found that feelings of being supported arise from an overall sense that the individual's pain and suffering matter to someone else whom he or she sees as significant or central to a support network (Remen 1991; Spiegel 1991, 1993; Cassell 1997; Chapman 1997). If stress levels decrease when an individual receives social support, then the opposite might also be true.

In a randomized, longitudinal study of eighty-six recurrent breast cancer patients, Spiegel showed that over time, pain and suffering increased in subjects assigned to a control group and decreased in subjects in the treatment group (Spiegel 1993). This study is of landmark importance, for several reasons: (1) the individuals in the treatment group lived 1.8 times longer than the controls; (2) it raised basic questions about the provider-patient relationships in medicine; and (3) it was one of the first longitudinal studies that highlighted the relevance of clinical and emotional support from the physician to the treatment of recurrent cancer patients (Spiegel 1993; Remen 1991). The implications of this study are also clearly relevant and applicable to other types of chronic illnesses and diseases.

Unfortunately, in underserved patient populations most interventions fail to respond to the needs for social, emotional, or clinical support (Ashing-Giwa et al. 1997). Ashing-Giwa and colleagues found that most African-American survivors receive information and support inadequate to help them through the initial diagnosis and treatment phases of the breast cancer experience. Moreover, many of the women, especially if they were poor, have no relationship with a primary care physician (Ashing-Giwa et al. 1997, 19–24).

The women in my study confirmed that social support (both direct and indirect) was an important channel through which they narrated life concerns. Their needs for social support were experienced across public and private domains. The significance of social support as a topic of discussion and as a social reality could be seen in their interpretations of their lives after breast cancer.

Another area that I found illuminating involved the ways the women talked about how they learned about new trends in cancer research. One common trend they spoke about was survivorship. Individuals in many cancer populations are now living longer. The main emphasis of many survivorship studies include (1) decreasing long and short-term psychological morbidity, (2) social support, (3) family, and (4) caring for the whole person in terms of quality of life. However, many of the women told me they felt that many of the current interventions designed by cancer organizations to help women cope with breast cancer overwhelmingly privilege white women's experience and coping with the disease, at the expense of African-American women.

The shifting sense of having cancer, of being deleted from survivorship, and assumptions about social support on a personal level meant that other aspects of the self needed to be reinterpreted as well. Most women believed that the experience of illness had transformed their lives and the way in which they interpreted their realities, their values, and their social relationships. Rather than experiencing the self as autonomous and alone, the women in this study resisted these biomedical discourses and reappraised the significance and the meanings of their experiences by pulling together to form a support group, one that was informed by their cultural experiences as African-American women who were coping with, and trying to survive, breast cancer. Those who did not belong to a support group that was predominantly African-American spoke in great detail about the need to start one. These women had made certain choices to speak and to act, while attempting to cope with overwhelming odds and the reality of death. Social support for these women began with and evolved from notions of extended kinship ties. Survival was linked to one's emotional and economic connectedness and to the embeddedness of these relations to biological kin, especially those who were also afflicted with breast cancer. For example, the women who were interviewed often described being extremely close to family members, even if no one knew they had cancer.

One woman, Cassandra Ewing, told me that her daughter "did not want to know [that she, Cassandra, had cancer] since she [the daughter] now had twin girls." It hurt Cassandra that her daughter did not want to know about the cancer, since she was only forty-seven and was Stage III. She somehow said, "I understand, I just hope that at some point she might hear me. We are still close and we talk about everything else but cancer. And I can understand that." Others told me that they went to the support group, since many daughters and other family members "might not want to know."

Others wanted life to go on as before for everyone else, since it was the sense of moving back to "life as before" that made one woman feel what she described as "alive and the same." The searches for social networks were motivated by the need to talk about cancer in an African-American public sphere. They were also inspired by the need to find sustenance in meaning making, an action enhanced by emotional connectedness to other survivors, to present concerns and everyday realities. While many had decided to disclose their cancer in the family and on the job, others had told no one but the women in the support group. One seventy-four year old grandmother, whom I will call Eugenia Edwards, told me:

Women just don't talk about that with men, or other people, just doctors.... Cancer is a private thing. I am still the same person. The only one who needs to know is the doctor and now these women. I do know how to ask for help now. Sometimes I get so tired and I need help with the groceries. That is something I had to learn.

Social support means different things to different people. On one level it is a symbol of the self, of ability to get assistance immediately when one needs it while maintaining a sense of independence. This is what some researchers have termed "functional support" (Smith 1995; Beattie 1997). For others, social support is a symbol of social and emotional relatedness to other people, and of the varying levels of involvement and the choices that one could make with respect—both to those who are significant and those who are marginal. Thus the significance and meanings of social support were intricately linked to an attempt to find meaning in the contexts of a woman's current life events, which included but were not limited to breast cancer. It was fundamental to the ways in which the woman perceived, experienced, and vocalized the emotional force of her life and her presence as a distinct self, embedded and defined in the context of social others, a sense that she was viable, of worth, and alive. In sum, perceptions of social support affected an individual's woman's life course and life force, and they influenced what she saw as her life choices.

In another interview in Houston I met Karen Tate, a fifty-three-year-old, Stage I, African-American breast cancer survivor who was interested in Tamoxifen. Karen told me about her experiences of feeling marginalized when she tried to find someone to show the women in the Sisters Network how to take care of themselves cosmetically after chemotherapy and radiation. The American Cancer Society has a program called "Look Good Feel Better." She told me about her dissatisfaction with their program:

That woman from that organization told us that we should be happy with [the makeup] we could get, but all the colors were for white or light skinned complexions and not for brown or dark skinned black women. Now why should we be happy with that? [Karen, June 1997].

In Karen's example the women decided to purchase makeup that would match their complexions. These narratives briefly highlight the surface details of breast cancer survivorship. These women consistently felt excluded from the ways survivorship had traditionally been constructed due to an insensitivity to their predicament as African-American breast cancer survivors. They were not alone; other women cited the popular literature on the subject. One woman told me that "a lot of the advertising on the subject has only white women on the cover and as models. I guess they just forget that we die too." Another woman after I had asked a question about how she felt about difficulty in getting a prosthesis in her skin color, looked at me directly and said in an almost scolding voice, "Are you really surprised that this happens to us? We are not important. It is their mothers and wives and daughter that matter, they will do all that it takes for them—and not us." I questioned her further to find out who the "them" was; and she replied, "Doctors, those in power, real power and big business."

Many of these issues might seem insignificant or even superficial to some people. But just imagine a cultural history of exclusion, where young African-American girls who are healthy are constantly assaulted by media that depict certain aspects of whiteness as beauty, femininity, and love (Morrison 1993; Hooks 1991; Davis 1994; Moore 1998). White women in this regard are perceived to be consistently embraced culturally, structurally, and emotionally when they are well. Moreover, they are culturally and clinically embraced in their experiences with this disease in ways that African-American women consistently are not. Indeed, it is well known among these women that in the public sphere of health and beauty, white women are consistently validated; it only makes sense that the experiences of white women who are breast cancer survivors would be validated long before those of African-American women are even considered. While cancer and certainly breast cancer is stigmatized, within this process there is a hierarchy, one that is reinforced through cultural practices and in institutions.

I came to understand the role of what Rosaldo has termed as *cultural force of emotion* and its relationship to bodily, self, and emotional experience and integrity. In his work among the Illogots of northern Luzon in the Philippines, Rosaldo (1993) stated, "The notion of force [in this instance life force] involved both affective intensity and significant consequences that unfold over a long period of time" (Rosaldo 1989, 20). It was in this manner, and from our conversations about breast cancer and life experiences, that I realized how perceptions about social support and inclusion are linked to the viability of life, emotional honesty, integrity, and life experiences, including breast cancer. Nonetheless, breast cancer is not ranked number one as a life focus. Social support and the perception that one is included and one can participate—actively make choices in the fight to survive, to overcome, and to live—became central experiential links between these African-American breast cancer survivors' ideas about what had caused their cancer, their experiences with what I call "uneven" care, and the context of everyday living.

This is a too-brief account of a myriad of experiences. By its brevity I do not mean to posit that there is an essential African-American female identity and experience. Rather, I am trying to show that in order to begin to understand the symbols and realities that underlie biomedicine's relationship to African-American women with breast cancer, we must understand the economic, historical, and cultural factors and lenses that situate these life experiences.

CONCLUSIONS

This chapter began as my attempt to gain some insight into the rather disturbing phenomenon of differential mortality in white and African-American women with breast cancer in the United States. I decided to examine the issue of differential mortality by emphasizing the link between perceived discrimination in the primarily biomedical encounters and the cultural effects of these perceptions on these participants, experiences of health, illness, and looking death in the face.

Only very recently have the metaphor and reality of cancer become one, evoking in survivors and in those who around them images of fear, suffering, agonizing pain, debilitating illness, and a brutal extinguishing of one's present reality. However, contemporary biomedical discourses about cancer have recently presented cancer in a new form, as a possibly curable, and for many a survivable, disease (Wingo et al. 1998). Such shifts in cognition and the meanings attached to cancer take time, but in the public arena, survivorship is the new ball game. A variety of tools, such as social support, enhance one's ability to win in the new game.

On the other hand, there has recently been shocking news in the breast cancer literature about decreased survival from breast cancer in African-American women. Articles have highlighted possible biological mechanisms influencing disease progression, such as estrogen receptor status, or the possibility of more aggressive tumors in younger women (Gastur et al. 1996). Even more recent discussions have attempted to take social and environmental factors into account in understanding why this sad phenomenon persists (Freeman 1998). Unfortunately, all we get is a "why," which when linked to the repeated affirmation in a public discourse of cancer "cures or survival," sounds more and more like a death knell to African-American breast cancer survivors. The answer to the knell is always the same—nobody knows. Thus, these women's experiences are often relegated to the back burner. While there has been a heightened awareness of cancer in the broad sense of media attention, there is still an overwhelming silence that surrounds many African-American women's discussions of this experience.

Other writers have also noted this silence. Before her death in 1991, Audre Lorde (1984), an African-American poet, author, and breast cancer survivor, addressed the relationships between gender, race, illness, and health. She argued the necessity for activism and a removal of the silence that often codes the language in which people speak about cancer. Such silences have also been used (often ineffectively) as a method to wage war against disease (Sontag 1979). Lorde believed that we need to counteract these silences with knowledge and activism. She maintained that breast cancer activism is necessary for the empowerment of women, African-American women in particular. She claimed:

The quality of light by which we scrutinize our lives has direct bearing upon the product, which we live, and upon the changes, which we hope to bring in our lives. It is within this light that we form those ideas by which we pursue our magic and make it realized. But for women living within structures defined by profit, by linear power, by institutional dehumanization, our feelings were not meant to survive. Moreover it is experience that has taught us that action in the now is also necessary, always. (Lorde 1984, 38–39)

The time for action, knowledge, and understanding is now.

ACKNOWLEDGMENTS

This chapter was supported by NIH grant 2HSA423. I want to thank the following people for their helpful suggestions: my mentor David Spiegel, M.D., professor in the Psychiatry Department at Stanford University, while I was a postdoctoral fellow in the Department of Psychiatry and Behavioral Sciences at Stanford Medical Center; Frank Staggers, M.D., Medical Director of the Haight–Ashbury Clinic in San Francisco; Diane Weiner, Ph.D.; Lee O. Carter, Jr., Annell Williams, Juanita Moore; Precilla Banks, Pamela Priest-Nave, M.A., Robert Hyiatt, M.D., Ph.D., and Rena Pasick, Ph.D., at the Northern California Cancer Center in Union City, California, and N. Bryant of Oakland, California, for their suggestions. Of course, I take responsibility for all interpretations that are made in this chapter.

LITERATURE CITED

American Cancer Society. 1997. *Cancer facts 1997*. Atlanta, GA.

Ansell, D., et al. 1993. Race, income and survival from breast cancer at two public hospitals. *Cancer* 72:2974–2978.

Asbury, Charles A. 1994. Psychosocial, cultural, and accessibility factors associated with participation of African-Americans in rehabilitation. *Rehabilitation Psychology* 39(2):113–121.

Ashing-Giwa, K., et al. 1997. Understanding the breast cancer experience of African-American women. *Journal of Psychosocial Oncology* 15(2):19–35.

Becker, A. E. 1995. *Body, self, and society: The view from Fiji.* Philadelphia: University of Pennsylvania Press.

Beisecker, A., M. Brecheisen, J. Ashworth, and J. Hayes. 1996. Older persons' medical encounters and their outcomes. *Research on Aging* 18(1):9–31.

—. 1996. Perceptions of the role of cancer patients' companions during medical appointments. *Journal of Psychosocial Oncology* 14(4):29–45.

Bradburn, J. et al. 1995. Developing clinical trial protocols: The use of patient focus groups. *Psycho-Oncology.* 4:107–112.

Byrd, W. M., and Linda A. Clayton. 1993. The African-American cancer crisis: A prescription. *Journal of Health Care for the Poor and Underserved* 4(2):102–116.

Carby, H. 1987. *Reconstructing womanhood.* New York: Oxford University Press.

Cassell, E. J. 1997. The nature of suffering and the goals of medicine. In *The Social Medicine Reader,* ed. Henderson et al., 13–22. Durham, NC: Duke University Press.

Catalan, J., A. Burgess, A. Pergami, and N. Hulme. 1996. The psychological impact on staff of caring for people with serious diseases: The case of HIV infection and oncology. *Jornal of Psychosomatic Research* 40(4):425–435.

Chapman, H. A., S. E. Hobfoll, and C. Ritter. 1997. Partners' stress underestimations lead to women's distress: A study of pregnant inner city women. *Journal of Personality and Social Psychology* 73(2):418–425.

Chevarley, F., and E. White. 1997. Recent trends in breast cancer mortality among white and black U.S. women. *American Journal of Public Health* 87(5):775–781.

Comaroff, J. 1984. Medicine, time and the perception of death. *Listening: Journal of Religion and Culture* 19:155–169.

Curbow, B., and M. R. Somerfield. 1995. Psychosocial resource variables in cancer studies: Conceptual and measurement issues: Introduction. (Special Issue)—Psychosocial resource variables in cancer studies: Conceptual and measurement issues. *Journal of Psychosocial Oncology* 13(1–2):1–9.

Davis, A. 1990. Sick and tired of being sick and tired: The politics of black women's health. In *The black women's health book: Speaking for ourselves,* ed. E C. White, 18–26. Seattle: Seal.

—. 1994. Surrogates and outcast mothers: Racism and reproductive politics. In *It just ain't fair: The ethics of health care for African-Americans,* ed. Annette Dula and Sara Goering, 41–56. Westport, CT: Praeger.

Descartes, R. 1960. *Meditations of first philosophy.* Trans. Laurence Lafleur. New York: Bobbs-Merrill.

Dressler, W. W. 1990. Lifestyle, stress and blood pressure in a southern black community. *Psychosomatic Medicine* 7:259–275.

Duelberg, Sonja I. 1992. Preventive health behavior among black and white women in urban and rural areas. *Social Science & Medicine* 34(2):191–198.

Eagleton, T. 1991. *Ideology: An introduction.* London, New York: Verso.

—. 1982. *The Rape of Clarissa.* Oxford: Basil Blackwell.

Eley J. W., et al. 1994. Racial differences in survival from breast cancer. *Journal of the American Medical Association* 272:947–954.

Epps, C. 1990. On conjuring cancer. In *The black women's health book: Speaking for ourselves,* ed. E. C. White, 38–43. Seattle: Seal.

Fanon, Frantz. 1968. *The Wretched of the Earth.* New York: Grove.

Fawzy, F., N. W. Fawzy, L. A. Arndt, and R. O. Pasnau. 1995. Critical review of psychosocial interventions in cancer care. *Archives of General Psychiatry* 1995(52):100–110.

Fawzy, F., N. W. Fawzy, C. S Hyun, and R. Elashoff. 1993. Malignant melanoma: Effects of an early structured psychiatric intervention, coping and affective state of recurrence and survival 6 years later. *Archives of General Psychiatry* 50:681–689.

Fox, H. E., S. A. White, M. H. F. Kao, R. Fernald, and D. Russell. 1997. Stress and dominance in a social fish. *Journal of Neuroscience.* 17(16):6463–6469.

Fraser, Nancy. 1990. *Rethinking the public sphere: A contribution to the critique of actually existing democracy.* Milwaukee: University of Wisconsin-Milwaukee, Center for Twentieth Century Studies.

Freeman, H. P. 1998. The meaning of race in science-considerations for cancer research. *Cancer* 82:219–225.

Friedman, L. et al. 1996. Early breast cancer detection behaviors among ethnically diverse low income women. *Psycho-Oncology* 5:283–289.

Gamble, V. 1989. *Germs have no color lines: Blacks and American medicine, 1900–1940,* ed. Vanessa Northington Gamble. New York: Garland.

—. 1990. On becoming a physician: A dream not deferred. In *The black women's health book: Speaking for ourselves,* ed. E. C. White, 52–64. Seattle: Seal.

Gapstur, S. M., et al. 1996. Hormone receptor status of breast tumors in black, Hispanic and non-Hispanic white women. *Cancer* 77:1465–1471.

Glanz, K., and C. Lerman. 1992. Psychosocial impact of breast cancer: A critical review. *Annals of Behavioral Medicine* 14(3):204–212.

Goffman, E. 1963. *Stigma: Notes on management of spoiled identity.* Englewood Cliffs, NJ: Prentice-Hall.

Gordon, D. 1990. Embodying illness, embodying culture. *Culture, Medicine, and Psychiatry,* 14(2):275–297.

Gregg, J., and R. H. Curry. 1994. Explanatory models for cancer among African-American women at two Atlanta neighborhood health centers: The implications for a cancer screening program. *Social Science and Medicine* 39(4):519–526.

Gutman, H. G. 1976. *The black family in slavery and freedom, 1750–1925.* New York: Vintage Books.

Habermas, J. 1984. *Theory of communicative action.* Boston: Beacon.

Hahn, R. A, ed. 1985. *Physicians of western medicine: Anthropological approaches to theory and practice.* Dordrecht, Boston: D. Reidel.

Heinrich, R. L., and C. Schag. 1987. The psychosocial impact of cancer: Cancer patients and healthy controls. *Journal of Psychosocial Oncology* 5(3):75–91.

Janz, N., and M. Becker. 1984. The health belief model: A decade later. *Health Education Quarterly* 11(1):1–47.

Jones, L., ed. 1989. *Minorities and cancer.* New York: Springer-Verlag.

Jones, J. H. 1993. *Bad blood: The Tuskegee syphilis experiment.* New York: Free Press.

Josefson, D. 1998. Breast cancer trial stopped early (editorial). *British Medical Journal* 316:1185.

Kaplan, S., et al. 1989. Assessing the effects of physician-patient interactions on the outcomes of chronic disease: erratum. *Medical Care* 27(7):679.

King, A. 1993. The impact of incarceration on African-American families: Implications for practice. *Families in Society* 74(3):145–153.

Kleinman, A. 1995. *Writing at the margin: Discourse between anthropology and medicine.* Berkeley: University of California Press.

Krieger, N., and S. Sidney. 1996. Racial discrimination and blood pressure: The CARDIA study of young black and white adults. *American Journal of Public Health* 86(10):1370–1378.

Landes, J. 1988. *Women and the public sphere in the age of the French Revolution.* Ithaca, NY: Cornell University Press.

Landrine, H., and E. A. Klonoff. 1996. The schedule of racist events: A measure of racial discrimination and a study of its negative physical and mental health consequences. *Journal of Black Psychology* 22(2):144–168.

Lerman, C., et al. 1993a. Communication between patients with breast cancer and health care providers: Determinants and implications. *Cancer* 72(9):2612–2620.

Lerman, C. et al. 1993b. Mammography adherence and psychological distress among women at risk for breast cancer. *Journal of the National Cancer Institute* 85(13):1074–1080.

Lock, M., and D. Gordon, eds. 1988. *Biomedicine examined.* Dordrecht and Boston: Kluwer.

Lorde, A. 1984. *Sister outsider: Essays and speeches.* Freedom, CA: Crossing.

——. 1980. *The cancer journals.* San Francisco: Aunt Lute.

Love, S. (with Karen Lindsey). 1995. 2d. ed. *Dr. Susan Love's breast book.* New York: Addison-Wesley.

Mathews, H., D. R. Lannin, and J. P. Mitchell. 1994. Coming to terms with advanced breast cancer: Black women's narratives from eastern North Carolina. *Social Science & Medicine* 38(6):789–800.

McGann, K. P. 1994. Sex bias in the treatment of coronary artery disease: Equity and quality of care. *Journal of Family Practice* 39(4):327–329.

Middlebrook, C. 1996. *Seeing the crab: A memoir of dying.* New York: Basic Books.

Moore, R. J. 1988. Mass media and Culture: African-American women and disordered eating. (under review).

——. 1997. Bonding with pain. Ph.D. Dissertation, Stanford University.

——. 1998. Black women, spirituality and breast cancer. Unpublished manuscript.

Morrison, T. 1993. *The bluest eye.* New York: Knopf.

Mosteller, F., and D. P. Moynihan, eds. 1972. *On equality of educational opportunity.* New York: Random House.

Moyinhan, D. 1965. *The negro family: The case for national action.* United States Labor Department: Office of Policy Planning and Research.

Murphy, G., L. B. Morris, and D. Lange. 1997. *Informed decisions: The complete book of cancer diagnosis, treatment and recovery.* New York: Viking Penguin.

Omalade, B. 1983. Hearts of darkness. In *Powers of desire: The politics of sexuality,* ed. Ann Snitow, Christine Stansell, and Sharon Thompson, 350–370. New York: Monthly Review.

Omi, M., and H. Winant. 1994. *Racial formation in the United States: From the 1960s to the 1990s.* New York: Routledge.

Penn, N., et al. 1995. Panel VI: Ethnic minorities, health care systems, and behavior. *Health Psychology* 14(7):641–646.

Pham, C. T., and S. J. McPhee. 1992. Knowledge, attitudes and practices of breast and cervical screening among Vietnamese women. *Journal of Cancer Education* 7(4):305–310.

Proctor, R. 1995. *Cancer wars: How politics shapes what we know and don't know about cancer.* New York: Basic Books.

Ries L. A., et al. 1994. *SEER cancer statistics review, 1973–1991: Tables and graphs.* Bethesda, MD: National Cancer Institute.

Remen, R. N. 1991. Working the gray zone: The dilemma of the private practitioner. *Advances* 7(3):36–40.

Rosaldo, M. 1980. *Knowledge and passion*. London: Cambridge University Press.

Rosaldo, R. 1993. *Culture and truth: The remaking of social analysis*. Boston: Beacon Press.

Sapolsky, R. M. 1994. *Why zebras don't get ulcers*. New York: W. H. Freeman.

Schneider, D. 1984. *A critique of the study of kinship*. Ann Arbor: University of Michigan Press.

Silverman, K. 1983. *The subject of semiotics*. New York: Oxford University Press.

Smith. M. 1995. Unmet needs for help among persons with AIDS. *AIDS Care* 7(3):353–363.

Sontag, S. 1979. *Illness as metaphor*. New York: Vintage Books.

Spiegel, D. 1993. *Living beyond limits: New hope and health for facing life-threatening illness*. New York: Time Books.

—. Cancer and depression. *British Journal of Psychiatry* 168(30):109–116.

—. 1996. Psychosocial influences on cancer incidence and progression. *Harvard Review of Psychiatry* 4(1):10–26.

Spiegel, D., and R. J. Moore. 1997. Imagery and hypnosis in the treatment of cancer patients. *Oncology* 11(8):1179–1190.

Stack, C. 1974. *All our kin: Strategies for survival in a black community*. New York: Harper and Row.

Staggers, F., C. Alexander, and K. Walton. 1990. Importance of reducing stress and strengthening the host in drug detoxification: The potential offered by transcendental meditation. Special Double Issue: Self-recovery: Treating addictions using transcendental meditation and Maharishi Ayur-Veda: II. *Alcoholism Treatment Quarterly* 11(3-4):297–331.

Stahly, G. 1988. Psychosocial aspects of the stigma of cancer: An overview. *Journal of Psychosocial Oncology* 6(3/4):3–27.

Staples, R., ed. 1993. Black families at the crossroads: Challenges and prospects. San Francisco: Jossey-Bass.

Taylor-Gibbs, J., et al. ed. 1988. Young, black, and male in America: An endangered species. Dover, MA: Auburn House.

Van Dulmen, A. M., J. F. M. Fennis, H. G. A. Mokkink, and H. G. M. van der Velden. 1995. Doctor-dependent changes in complaint-related cognitions and anxiety during medical consultations in functional abdominal complaints. *Psychological Medicine* 25(5):1011–1018.

Wingo, P., L. Ries, H. Rosenberg, D. Miller, and B. Edwards. 1998. Cancer incidence and mortality, 1973-1995: A report card for the U.S. *Cancer* 82(6):1197–1207.

Wojcik, B. E., M. A. Spinks, and S. A. Optenberg. 1998. Carcinoma survival analysis for African-American and white women in an equal-access health care system. *Cancer* 82:1310–1318.

Chapter 5

American Indian Cancer Discourse and the Prevention of Illness

Diane Weiner

Health providers trained in biomedicine assert that talking and thinking about cancer are critical to cancer prevention, detection, and care. However, many lay people in North America and elsewhere attribute the onset of cancer to thinking about and discussing this condition. What are the roots of this conflict? As importantly, what impact do these differences have on cancer prevention and control? In this chapter, I provide a sociocultural analysis of American Indian cancer discourse patterns as an example of the ways in which people attempt to prevent the onset of cancer. Distinct cultural-discourse approaches represent one method.

Historically, many American Indians have viewed health as a harmonious connection between body, mind, and spirit.[1] Culturally appropriate actions are felt to bring well-being (see Lake 1982; Adair et al. 1988; Trafzer 1997), while balance between an individual and his/her secular and spiritual surroundings prevents illness (see Beck and Walters 1977; Locust 1986; Molina 1997). Many contemporary individuals share these convictions (see Black Feather 1992; Loftin 1994, 649). Though diverse and dynamic, American Indian and Alaska Native prevention methods invoke personal and collective means of protection (Joe 1994). Reflecting other life patterns, individual wellness is thought to enhance the overall health of a community.

Ideas about causation and prevention may influence and in turn be influenced by cancer detection and treatment practices. People may tie distinct etiologic beliefs to particular treatment methods. Lay individuals may associate certain life-threatening conditions, such as tuberculosis (Adair et al. 1988) or cancer, with more than one etiology (see Csordas 1989; Colomeda 1996; see also Chavez et al. 1995). Care for both causes may be sought. An American Indian female cancer survivor with whom I spoke stated that certain cancers may be provoked by both "evil thoughts" and "genetic inheritance," making both tribal prayers and genetic testing appropriate prevention methods. These different techniques may be used sequentially or simultaneously. This woman had used prayer throughout her life— sometimes before, during, or after clinical procedures. She was praying not in or- der to influence a clinical outcome but rather for spiritual assistance to dispell ill- ness-causing malevolence. She also consulted geneticists and physicians. Like other people in her community who embraced more than one religion (native and Catholic, native and Protestant), she compartmentalized distinct beliefs and be- haviors about health (see also Strickland et al. 1996).

The use of indigenous and biomedical health systems is not unique to American Indians. Indeed the employment of multiple health systems, especially by people who are enduring chronic or life-threatening illnesses, is common (see Kleinman 1980, 1988; Young 1982; Scrimshaw 1992).

Among certain tribes and individuals, prevention involves the purification of thoughts so that certain maladies, including cancer, are neither mentioned nor contemplated (Cobb 1996; Burhansstipanov 1997). Indeed, among the Diné (Na- vajo), thinking or speaking about an illness may cause its onset or the destruction of entire communities (Levy et al. 1987; see also Antle 1987). Moreover, those who speak about or diagnose cancer are felt to have the power of condemnation— this view about cancer is widespread (Gordon 1990; Gordon and Paci 1997). These ideas about the power of words may derive from notions of purity and pol- lution that classify words or thoughts as positive or negative (see Douglas 1966). Naming a problem or an illness lends weight to its existence, such that a diagnosis of or remark about cancer changes this word from a concept or possibility to an actual or remembered reality, one associated with fear, pain, and mortality (see Favret-Saada 1980, Coutin 1995).

For adherents to these views, clinical cancer prevention practices may be foresworn, or pose dilemmas. An understanding of the social context in which "cancer talk" appears to be avoided is necessary if cancer prevention and control practitioners and advocates are to develop culturally sensitive prevention and de- tection strategies. In the next few pages, I will review underlying factors that influ- ence speech about illness. Case studies illustrate who may and may not object to a public or private discussion of cancer. I will assess several etiologic, diagnostic, sociodemographic, linguistic, cultural, and religious reasons for these feelings. This information provides a framework for an examination of the practical implications for health promotion and care.

ETIOLOGY OF CANCER TALK

Qualitative anthropological studies that I conducted among members of four American Indian tribes in southern California reveal that for them, discussing lung, colon, breast, and cervical cancers does not appear to invite disaster. This stance seems to resemble that of the Inuit women of Labrador and the Inupiat women of Alaska interviewed by Lorelei Colomeda during the 1990s. These women do not seem to display concern about discussions of cancer (Colomeda 1996).

The southern Californian Indians whom I interviewed considered different types of cancer to have multiple etiologies. Like other illnesses, cancer was attributed to the actions of a human or an object, such as a gene. Those who believe that genes cause cancer view genes as inseparable from the whole body. One female cancer survivor commented on this idea, asking, "How could it [the body] be separate? Genes are what make us" (Weiner 1997).

Most interviewees did not consider cancer to be inevitably terminal. Preliminary analysis of informal interviews with fifty-one adults illustrated that all but one had met or heard of a cancer survivor. Indeed, twelve individuals had a history of one or more cancers, and four others had had benign tumors. Thirty-one people had a family member or close friend with a history of cancer. Four others "knew of" people who had this condition. Cancer is known to and discussed among members of native populations of southern California. At least during this decade, cancer diagnoses have rarely been deliberately kept secret from family members. In contrast, during the 1950s, 1960s, and 1970s individuals were less apt to discuss cancer diagnoses with other lay people, although relatives linked the deaths of those who had been ill to cancer.

One breast cancer survivor remarked that "some people" still, generally unsuccessfully, "try to hide" diagnoses of cancer. This woman stated that cancer is not "an illness to be ashamed of—you just do something about it—you can't help it if you got it." When I inquired why might people be ashamed, this woman corrected herself and claimed, "Actually I think they're in shock". After this shock subsides, cancer patients purportedly act.

The recent "openness" regarding cancer reporting may be more common in relatively small communities, in which individuals who are ill or undergoing care are: (1) missed at such events as work, school, or meetings; (2) seen by others at local or municipal treatment facilities; (3) subjects of gossip; (4) visibly changed; or (5) under the care of other community members. Furthermore, these people are later seen and met with after treatments conclude. Increasingly, cancer is a public affair (Weiner 1993, 1997).

American Indians of southern California do not perceive cancer to be spread through talk. Etiologies generally include dietary, genetic, and environmental sources. Three out of thirty-six women interviewed felt that breast cancers among older women may be a result of past improper breast-feeding habits and poor hygiene. These women learned about these improprieties from popular and clinical health practices. Interviewees also reported learning about cancers through television, popular magazines, health education literature, conversations with medical personnel, clergy, other tribal members (especially sisters and mothers), friends, observations of those with cancer, and tribal oral histories. The majority of this information is passed in English.

Some male and female cancer patients of different ages, religious affiliations (Protestant, Catholic, or native), and tribal backgrounds assert that cancer may be caused by evil thoughts, either accidental or intentional. Such thoughts may be initiated by the eventual victim or by a person who sends these bad feelings to someone else (Weiner 1997).

Camille, a cancer survivor, has had several bouts with cancer and with benign tumors throughout her life. She understands a few words of her native language, but like most of her reservation "age mates" she can not hold a conversation in this language. She once was told by another tribal member that cancer in a person's body may be initiated by evil within that person. Camille does not agree with this statement and claims to have made no efforts to change her ways on that basis. Since childhood, Camille has continued to obtain assistance through clinical means and the Catholic Church.

Edith, another cancer survivor, resides on a neighboring reservation and is fluent in her native language and in English. She does not think that there is a word for cancer in her native tongue; instead one would use the word for "feeling bad," or "not well." According to Edith, cancer is an "ugly disease, a painful disease." She asserts that the "negativity and evil thoughts or feelings" of others caused her different cancers. Edith countered these thoughts and accompanying illnesses through the use of several health methods: clinical cancer care, Christian prayer, indigenous therapies, and personal fortitude. She remarks, "Mentally I refused, I refused death, I refused sickness, I was determined my body was going to be all right."

THOUGHTS AND POWER

The view that malevolent persons may cause maladies in other peoples' bodies is echoed by members of many California tribes. Beings can create and send power. Those who have such powers are rare but dangerous. They may hide from others (Bean 1976, 1992; Walker and Hudson 1993). Dialogues with such individuals may or may not disclose their bad intentions. Among southern California American Indians, discussions of cancer in a social, clinical, anthropological, or research context by those *without* bad intentions do not seem associated with the onset of this illness. For the most part, such people are easily identified.

PHILOSOPHICAL SOURCES

Like those of primordial beings depicted in American Indian oral narratives, the actions of contemporary native people seem to be on the level of thoughts rather than of words. In a religious context, language, spoken or silent, aids in the creation (and continuation) of the universe. More often than not, American Indian worlds are caused or molded by thinking rather than by speaking. For instance, the Diegueño (Waterman 1910), Diné (Navajo) (see Witherspoon 1977), and Apache deities thought the world into existence. Among the Zuni (Tedlock 1972) and Achumawi and Atsugawi (or Pit River) (Woiche 1992), primordial beings also shaped the world through their thoughts. Certain creators, like those of the Mohawk (Akweks n.d.), think about and then physically construct or manipulate the world. These thoughts of creation are revealed through stories, songs, chants, and prayers. Creation is not static; the stories, songs, chants, and prayers explain creation, but with every retelling, resinging, and repraying, the world is recreated anew. When performed in a ritual context, some ceremonial songs not only repeat the cycle of creation, but enable the world to be reborn or continue (Tedlock 1983). Thus, thoughts provide the impetus for phenomenological actions.

In a similar vein, according to many traditional American Indian philosophies, the thoughts of a human, garnered through observations of and interactions with others, influence his/her health as well as that of others (See Epple et al. 1997; Trafzer 1998). Being unique, individuals understand and manage distinct types of knowledge and power. Therefore, certain persons are potentially more able to affect well-being than are others (see Bean 1976, 1992; Morrison 1992).

Euro-American and Judeo-Christian concepts of thought and power have different roots. The Egyptian god Ptah created everything by speaking. The first three verses of the book of Genesis reminds Jews (and Christians) that to speak may be to create. After contact with Greeks (approximately 300 B.C.) and in particular with the theories of Plato, who argued that all existence has a form derived from an ideal, eternal form—Jews adopted the belief that the word is an extension of thought. Later, Christians claimed that "Jesus is the Word," a concept prefigured in the *Book of Wisdom*, a deutero-canonical writing of the Old Testament. In that text, wisdom represents not only the "Word" but also "the perfection of knowledge showing itself in action" (Gigot 1997). Notions about speech became even more intertwined with ideas concerning thought. Medieval Christian thinkers held that eternal ideas are in the mind of God. They argued that the world, in nature and art, imitates these thoughts and that the most a human can do is to try to mirror divine deliberations. In this view, thought at its highest reflects the eternal ideas in the mind of God (Weiner 1998). Thoughts, gazes, and words may influence one's health or that of others. For example, the "evil eye," arising from the jealousy of one person, can provoke ill health in another person. Prayer, both aloud and silent, may cause a saint to intercede in favor of an individual.

Western nineteenth-century idealistic philosophies and twentieth-century New Age thinking, perhaps outgrowths of Kant's writings, also assert that individuals may think reality into existence. Contemporary New Age and New Thought religions imply that positive thinking is healthy, while negative thinking is damaging (see Morrish 1998).

Some people feel that human thoughts impact only the thinker's condition (Townsend 1978). Others argue that thoughts may affect not only onself but others as well. Gordon and Paci point out that Italian doctors may deem discussed emotions to be "contagious" (Gordon and Paci 1997, 1441). U.S. medical professionals, such as Andrew Weil, also may assert that positive *thoughts* in association with actions may enable healing processes (Weil 1995; Kleinman 1988).

In sum, for followers of distinct religions and philosophical teachings, human deliberations in thought or speech can be powerful and even dangerous. Uncontrolled or malevolent thoughts may provoke illnesses. Such views appear to influence even the most seemingly secular or positivist persons (see Favret-Saada 1980). It may be that God, the First Beings, or other deities who have the ability to initiate beneficial or destructive actions are listening to humans. As Bruce Allen, Jr. notes, many African-American people feel that human thoughts and speech may waken the deities and cause them to act upon our ideas (Allen 1998).

AVOIDING TALK ABOUT ILLNESS

Members of different American Indian ethnic groups throughout the Southwest attempt to prevent cancer by avoiding discussion of certain aspects of this condition. These ethnicities embrace different language families (Athabascan, Uto-Aztecan), language isolates (Keresan), and geographic environments (mountains, plateaus, valleys). Importantly, not all groups nor individuals from the Southwest adhere to this policy. Giuliano and colleagues were able to conduct face-to-face interviews with 535 self-identified Hopi women (Hopi is part of the Uto-Aztecan language family) about breast and cervical cancer (Giuliano et al. 1998). This study indicates that these women discussed cancer with health care researchers.

Nonetheless, some individuals assert that to name a condition is to invite it into your body or into that of a listener. Others feel that thoughts on a subject may be equally influential. Women aged fifty years and older that I interviewed from one Southwestern group, tended to dodge public and personal conversations about the etiologies and symptoms associated with benign and malignant cervical and breast growths. Avoidance of this topic is facilitated by the common use of the term "tumors" to describe all growths in the body.

Prevention and treatment practices are more willingly described. For example, methods of cleaning one's breasts to prevent health problems are readily addressed. Screening programs, such as mammograms, and surgical treatment methods may also be mentioned. Interestingly, naming and discussing other illnesses perceived to be chronic or life threatening, such as Type 2 diabetes or AIDS, are not considered dangerous for dialogue participants.

Older men also seem at ease discussing the purported causes of prostate, colon, lung, and breast cancers, as well as of leukemia. These illnesses are all deemed to be deadly. All of the male speakers interviewed knew of someone affected by one or more of these conditions. They link the onset of prostate and colon cancers to consuming alcohol and tobacco and to leading a sedentary lifestyle. Lung cancer is tied to smoking habits. According to these retired miners and agricultural laborers, these cancers are also created by pesticides and other air and water-borne contaminants (Weiner 1996).

Women who have initiated one-on-one conversations or are willing to participate in group discussions about "tumors" of the breast and other sites tend to believe that these problems are treatable. These women know people who died from other types of tumors; they also each knew people who have survived "breast tumors" due to "lumpectomies and other surgeries." These women also claim to have participated in two different tribally sponsored health promotion programs in which women's health issues were discussed. Although "tumors" may be deemed treatable, when I asked one woman, "What if somebody doesn't get treated for it?" she murmured, "Hmmm," looked away, and did not respond. This reaction is not atypical. People may not talk about an extraordinary crisis condition that they wish to prevent.

SOME FACTORS THAT AFFECT TALK

During one group interview on the subject of "women's health," sixteen women participated. All of these women knew each other and had known me for thirteen months. The only person new to the group was a female anthropologist from a local university; the new anthropologist was, with the approval of the group, taking notes. After talking about other topics, including ways to detect breast tumors, the women were asked to describe the possible causes of cervical cancer. When I asked one woman, "Are there things, in your opinion, that might cause cervical cancer?" the woman next to her shouted, "She doesn't know and she doesn't want to know!" All the women in the room laughed in agreement. I then inquired, "If we don't want to know about what causes this, are there ways to prevent this?" Immediately responses rang out, both in the form of inquiries and declarative statements, leading to a five-woman discussion of postpartum health practices learned from sisters and mothers. These modes of prevention reportedly help to protect a woman from maladies and early death, since they focus on the genesis and etiologies of possible future problems.

Kira, whose mother died of cancer, argues that

some of the people, when it comes to this type of thing, they're very shy—that's the one thing about it, they're very very shy. I'm an out-going person, so when you mention something like [breast tumors] I find out about something like that. I always ask things.

Why are some people, as Kira says, "shy"?

Age may be a factor, especially in association with language use, religious beliefs, and gender. Felicia Hodge, along with her research team from the Center for American Indian Research and Education (Berkeley, California), interviewed northern Californian Indian women and members of several tribes relocated to the San Francisco Bay area about breast and cervical cancers. The women, all between the ages of eighteen and thirty, frequently claimed that their parents and grandparents had neither known the words for cancer nor had been willing to discuss this topic. The younger women were open to such conversations; these women did not associate cancer with "something bad you did" (Hodge 1998). Older women may be less willing to discuss issues concerning reproduction, associated body parts, and the illnesses that may attack them. As the women interviewed by Hodge and colleagues suggest, older women may be less likely to speak or think in English than in native languages that do not have words about cancer. The inability to name and as a result classify a condition may prevent a person from fully knowing its etiology and thus its accompanying cure (see also Favret-Saada 1980; Adair et al. 1988; Browner and Press 1996, 147).

In contrast to the case for people under forty-five years of age, English is not the primary language of anyone that I interviewed in the Southwest, other than Kira. The majority speak their native language or Spanish. The native language does not have words for cancer; no written cancer prevention materials exist in this language. Moreover, none of those interviewed who have received screening or treatment for themselves or family members claim to have interacted with physicians who spoke the clients' native language. Communication problems may arise due to misinterpretations, which may be exacerbated by anxieties concerning the illness and the hierarchical nature of doctor-patient communication practices (see West 1984; Todd 1993; Ubel 1995; Gordon and Paci 1997). Information may be missed, or it may be misunderstood. This situation is poignantly illustrated by Ava's description of her daughter's experience with leukemia. One day Ava and I discussed the possibility that leukemia is inherited. She said:

And I had a daughter, she was eighteen, when she died of leukemia, and what causes leukemia?

D: In your opinion, what causes this, leukemia?
Ava: I never knew, I used to wonder why she had leukemia, or where she got it. . . .
D: What did you do [when she was sick]? Did [the doctors] answer your questions?
Ava: No, they were asking me. The doctors were asking me, and I didn't know. When she was fifteen days old she was in the hospital for fifteen days in critical condition, and I never found out why, probably I didn't ask, that's why . . .
D: . . . Just in general why do you think cancer might happen? Just cancer in general, not leukemia?
Ava: I really don't know nothing about cancer.

Knowledge of clinical perspectives is uncommon among those interviewed. In contrast, lay cultural knowledge is shared.

One path of information is through religious activities. These women are apt to express openly both their native and Catholic religious beliefs. Several dictates concerning health are of consequence. First, a person may will a particular condition onto his/her self through thoughts of this malady. Second, illnesses may also develop if a person or a family member makes and then breaks a divine vow; retribution may be divinely meted out in the form of afflictions. Third, disruption of social rules may also cause harm to an individual or his/her family. Social transgressions by others (humans and spirits) may also be dangerous; it may be difficult to protect oneself from the malevolent thoughts or deeds of others. "Tumors" are associated with impurities and evil. Women may thus be susceptible to impurities that invite disaster.

A tribal physician from this community argues that according to many older tribal members, life-threatening womens' health problems are viewed as punishments for not practicing tribal postpartum health practices. Women from this group are thus held responsible for practicing cultural prevention methods in order to stay healthy in later years. Unfortunately, not all women perform these rituals, and some reportedly fear that they performed them improperly. Importantly, native and nonnative women throughout the United States have been taught to fear breast tumors as a possible result of improper social role maintenance. Popular health education campaigns urge that women who practice proper gender roles through child bearing and nursing are partially protected from breast cancer

(Reagan 1997); those who do not perform such practices place themselves in jeopardy.

The views of men contrast with those of older women. Men tend to link "tumors" to secular causes. Interestingly, although sedentary lifestyles are not considered by men to be behaviorally proper, other contributing factors to cancer (alcohol and commercial tobacco consumption, income-generating activities) are generally condoned among these older men. Discussion by men of health problems not tied to ritual nor sacred behaviors thus seems possible.

Like members of other groups (see Sontag 1978; Gregg and Curry 1994, 523), women of the Southwest tend to equate "tumors" with impending death. During interviews the women mention other women and children who have died from "tumors," leukemia, and other related conditions. Tribal health providers are cognizant of this "fear of cancer," surgeries, and "dying." As one local practitioner notes, "So many neighbors died of it" that those who fear that they might be ill "won't say anything 'til it's too late." This approach often perpetuates a cycle of mortality in which early clinical detection or treatment is deferred, and death occurs (see also Gregg and Curry 1994). One breast cancer survivor and public health educator who met with female community health workers of various ages discovered that they too associated breast tumors with death. The survivor later told the following story about such a meeting:

I'm here as a survivor and all I hear is death. Death sounds like all you know. Then a [tribal] survivor disclosed her breast cancer. Then another woman: endometrial. [This woman] felt she shouldn't get a hysterectomy and asked her priest for permission. Losing a body part tied to reproduction is a big thing. It's held in the family and that's all. More than diabetes, cancer equals death, not 'cause of the reality but because if it's only [discussed] with the family, immediate treatment is difficult. If you don't know somebody who survived, you skip the treatment.

Unlike people interviewed in California, these Southwestern women do not have much contact with cancer survivors. There is no legacy of hope, battle, or victory (see Patterson 1987; Good 1988; Good et al. 1990; Weiss 1997) associated with cancer among these older women. Upon contact with a breast cancer survivor, some women felt at ease talking about personal health conditions. This survivor and health educator emphasized that this discussion was a forum to provide clinical health information; tribal religious matters were not discussed.

"Tumors" in the breast and cervix among women of this tribe are often linked to improperly performed rituals or inappropriate thoughts. Acknowledgement of the former may leave one open to illness and social criticism. For instance, someone who admits having not participated in culturally preferred postpartum behaviors may be verbally admonished. This woman may also consider herself and be considered by her peers, to be a target for medical problems. This possibility may be strengthened if the woman feels that she might be receptive to malevolent musings. Discussions of etiologies and symptoms associated with "tumors" may include persons who consciously or unconsciously provoke ill will. Unlike divine beings, humans are not always able to know who harbors such thoughts. So women who are not "shy" may be susceptible to troubles.

Meira Weiss argues that "getting cancer [like heart disease or AIDS] is often understood as the fault of someone who has taken part in 'unsafe' behavior" (1997, 457). Those who acquire these medical problems are often perceived to be at fault. When associated with spiritual or religious etiologies, certain health conditions inspire not only fear of physical pain and death but also the anguish of social and spiritual pollution. Perhaps for this reason, families tend to work together to obtain divine forgiveness and assistance. One man from the Southwest told me that when a certain child had cancer, his family participated in many cultural activities. The family was, according to this man, "expecting God to make a miracle. This tends to make families more cohesive. They know the end result will be death, but they try and stop it. A miracle might happen so they made vows and [danced in ceremonies]."

The child eventually died, but the family members had had an opportunity to embrace one another, other community members, and God, socially, emotionally, spiritually, and culturally. Moreover, God had been offered prayers in the hopes of a cure for the child and absolution from any improprieties associated with his condition.

SUMMARY REMARKS

Discourse about cancer is influenced by several factors. Older individuals, especially those who have limited access to medical information in a familiar language, may have less opportunity and willingness to discuss clinically diagnosed diseases like cancer. Even though gender seems to play a key role in discourse strategies among members of certain tribes, men and women of southern California appear to use similar cancer discourse patterns.

Illnesses may seem more perilous if contact with those who have survived a condition is limited. Fear is compounded when information about efficacious therapies is unavailable or linguistically inaccessible. Clearly, ideas about cancer are greatly influenced by concepts of danger and stigma; however, the cultural and religious contexts for these differ. Clinical approaches suggest that secular behaviors may be tied to the advent of tumors, whereas some American Indian cultural approaches, especially among older Southwestern women interviewed, suggest that religious/spiritual actions are linked to the development of health problems.

Joshua, a California Indian elder, discussed this issue with me one night. He said, "Some people are not able to or privileged to understand certain things. Access to knowledge, to knowing, [things that are] dangerous could kill you." This man, who uses both tribal and clinical medicines for a chronic health ailment and speaks both English and his native language, believes that people of different backgrounds have distinct understandings of power.

Joshua is quite aware that for some people, ritual and secular health systems do not mix, cognitively or behaviorally (see also Csordas 1989). In California, multiple etiologies are attached to and enable distinct health behaviors. Some of these etiologies are linked to secular conditions. In other regions, this is not the case. For these reasons, individuals who withhold or appear to neglect knowledge or discussions of certain illnesses are practicing prevention as best as they know how. Most importantly, people who tend to avoid discussions of cancer symptoms, etiologies, and treatments are not necessarily in denial of their existence. What these people may need are (1) greater contacts with cancer survivors, (2) accessible information, and (3) culturally sensitive discussions framed in secular terms.

ACKNOWLEDGMENTS

Research for this paper was partially funded by the University of Arizona Cancer Epidemiology and Prevention Training Program and by the UCLA Institute of American Cultures. I am extremely grateful to all those who shared their stories about health with me. I wish to thank Susan Coutin, Paul Kroskrity, Rhonda Moore, Deena Newman, Clifford Trafzer, and Rob Weiner for their helpful comments.

NOTES

1. In this context, the term "American Indians" refers to the indigenous peoples of North America. The term "Native Americans" often includes American Indians, Alaska Natives, and native Hawaiians.

LITERATURE CITED

Adair, J., K. W. Dueuschle, and C. R. Barnett. 1988. *The people's health: Anthropology and medicine in a Navajo community.* Albuquerque: University of New Mexico Press.
Akweks, A. n.d. *Collection of Mohawk legends.* Onchiota, NY: Six Nations Indian Museum.
Allen, B. Jr. 1998, Personal communication, June.
Antle, A. 1987. Ethnic perspectives of cancer nursing: The American Indian. *Oncology Nursing Forum* 14(3):70–73.
Bean, L. J. 1976. Power and its applications in native California. In *Native Californians: A theoretical perspective*, ed. Lowell John Bean and Thomas C. Blackburn, 407–420. Socorro, NM: Ballena.
—. 1992. California Indian shamanism and folk curing. In *California Indian shamanism*, ed. Lowell John Bean, 53–66. Menlo Park, CA: Ballena.
Beck, P., and A. Walters. 1977. *The sacred; Ways of knowledge, sources of life.* Tsaile, AZ: Navajo Community College Press.
Black Feather, J. 1992. Cultural beliefs and understanding cancer. *American Indian Culture and Research Journal* 16(3):139–144.
Browner, C. H., and N. Press. 1996. The production of authoritative knowledge in American prenatal care. *Medical Anthropology Quarterly* 10(2):141–156.
Burhansstipanov, L. 1997. *Cancer among elder Native Americans.* Denver: University of Colorado, Health Sciences Center, National Center for American Indian and Alaska Native Mental Health Research.

Chavez, L., A. Hubbell, J. McMullin, R. Martinez, and S. Mishra. 1995. Understanding knowledge and attitudes about breast cancer: A cultural analysis. *Archives of Family Medicine* 4:145–152.

Cobb, N. 1996. Personal communication, December.

Colomeda, L. 1996. *Through the northern looking glass: Breast cancer stories told by northern native women.* New York: NLN.

Coutin, S. 1995. *The culture of protest: Religious activism and the U.S. sanctuary movement.* Boulder, CO: Westview.

Csordas, T. J. 1989. The sore that does not heal: Cause and concept in the Navajo experience of cancer. *Journal of Anthropological Research* 45:457–485.

DiGiacomo, S. 1987. Biomedicine as a cultural system: An anthropologist in the kingdom of the sick. In *Encounters with biomedicine: Case studies in medical anthropology,* ed. Hans Baer, 315–346. Philadelphia: Gordon and Breach.

Douglas, M. 1966. *Purity and danger: An analysis of concepts of pollution and taboo.* New York: Praeger.

Epple, C., F. Morgan, and M. Bauer. 1997. Implications of T'áá Hó Ájít'éego for Navajo diabetics. Society for Applied Anthropology Meetings, 7 March, Seattle, Washington.

Favret-Saada, J. 1980. *Deadly words.* Trans. Catherine Cullen. Cambridge: Cambridge University Press.

Garro, L. C., and G. C. Lang. 1994. Explanations of diabetes: Anishinaabeg and Dakota deliberate upon a new illness. In *Diabetes as a disease of civilization: The impact of lifestyle and cultural changes on the health of indigenous peoples,* ed. Jennie Joe and Rob Young, 293-328. Berlin: Mouton de Gruyter.

Gigot, F. E. 1997. Book of wisdom. In *The Catholic encyclopedia* [online]. Transcribed by Thomas M. Barret. Available: http://www.knight.org/advent/cathen/1566a.htm, 1998.

Giuliano, A., M. Papenfuss, J. de Guernsey de Zapien, S. Tilousi, and L. Nuvayestewa. 1998. Breast cancer screening among southwest American Indian women living on-reservation. *Preventive Medicine* 27:135–143.

Good, M. J. D. 1988. The practice of biomedicine and the discourse on hope. Paper presented at Anthropologies of Medicine, 4-8 December, Hamburg, Germany.

Good, M. J .D., B. Good, C. Schaffer, and S. Lind. 1990. American oncology and the discourse on hope. *Culture, Medicine, and Psychiatry* 14:59–79.

Gordon, D. 1990. Embodying illness, embodying culture. *Culture, Medicine, and Psychiatry* 14:275–297.

Gordon, D., and E. Paci. 1997. Disclosure practices and cultural narratives: Understanding concealment and silence around cancer in Tuscany, Italy. *Social Science and Medicine* 44(10):1433–1452.

Gregg, J., and R. Curry. 1994. Explanatory models for cancer among African-American women at two neighborhood health centers: The implications for a cancer screening program. *Medicine* 39:519–526.

Hodge, F. 1998. Personal communication, May.

Joe, J. 1994. Traditional health practices and cultural views. In *The native North American almanac,* ed. Duane Champagne, 801–811. Detroit: Gale Research.

Kleinman, A. 1980. *Patients and healers in the context of culture: An exploration of the borderland between anthropology, medicine, and psychiatry.* Berkeley: University of California Press.

—. 1988. *The illness narratives: Suffering, healing, and the human condition.* New York: Basic Books.

Lake, R., Jr. 1982. A discussion of Native American health problems, needs, and services with a focus on Northwestern California. *White Cloud Journal* 2(4):23–31.

Levy, J., R. Neutra, and D. Parker. 1987. *Hand trembling, frenzy witchcraft, and moth madness: A study of Navajo seizure disorders.* Tucson: University of Arizona Press.

Locust, C. 1986. *American Indian beliefs concerning health and unwellness.* Tucson: Native American Research and Training Center.

Loftin, J. 1994. Traditional religious practices among contemporary American Indians. In *The native North American almanac.* ed. Duane Champagne, 648–658. Detroit: Gale Research.

Molina, J. 1997. Cultural medicine. *Journal of Minority Medical Students* (Spring):28–32.

Morrish, J. 1998. These people believe positive thinking can cure cancer. *The Independent,* 5 July.

Patterson, J. T. 1987. *The dread disease: Cancer and modern American culture.* Cambridge, MA: Harvard University Press.

Reagan, L. J. 1997. Engendering the dread disease: Women, men, and cancer. *American Journal of Public Health* 87(11):1779–1787.

Scrimshaw, S. 1992. Adaptation of anthropological methodologies to rapid assessment of nutrition and primary health care. In *Rapid assessment procedures: Qualitative methodologies for planning and evaluation of health related programmes,* ed. Nevin S. Scrimshaw and Gary R. Gleason, 25–38. Boston: International Nutrition Foundation for Developing Countries.

Sontag, S. 1978. *Illness as metaphor.* New York: Farrar, Strauss, and Giroux.

Strickland, C. J., N. J. Chrisman, M. Yallup, K. Powell, and M. Dick Squeoch. 1996. Walking the journey of womanhood: Yakama Indian women and Papanicolaou (Pap) test screening. *Public Health Nursing* 13(2):141–150.

Tedlock, D., trans. 1972. *Finding the center: Narrative poetry of the Zuni Indians.* Lincoln: University of Nebraska Press.

—. 1983. The spoken word and the work of interpretation in American Indian religion. In *The spoken word and the work of interpretation,* ed. Dennis Tedlock, 233–246. Philadelphia: University of Pennsylvania Press.

Todd, A. D. 1993, 2nd ed. Exploring women's experiences: Power and resistance in medical discourse. In *The social organization of doctor-patient communication,* ed. Alexandra Dundas Todd and Sue Fisher, 267–285. Norwood, NJ: Ablex.

Townsend, J. 1978. *Cultural conceptions and mental illness: A comparison of Germany and America.* Chicago: University of Chicago Press.

Trafzer, C. E. 1997. Death stalks the Yakama. East Lansing: Michigan State University Press.

—. 1998. Personal communication, June.

Ubel, P. A. 1995. Doctor talk: Technology and modern conversation. *American Journal of Medicine* 98:587–588.

Walker, P. L. and T. Hudson. 1993. *Chumash healing: Changing health and medical practices in an American Indian society.* Banning, CA: Malki Museum Press.

Waterman, T. T. 1910. The religious practices of the Diegueño Indians. *University of California Publications in American Archaeology and Ethnology* 8(6):271–358.

Weil, A. 1995. *Spontaneous healing.* New York: Knopf.

Weiner, D. 1993. Dissertation field notes.

—. 1996. Postdoctoral field notes.

—. 1997. *Southern California Indian cancer prevention: Belief systems, support networks, and treatments,* field notes.

Weiner, R. 1998. Personal communication, June.

Weiss, M. 1997. Signifiying the pandemics: Metaphors of AIDS, cancer, and heart disease. *Medical Anthropology Quarterly* 11(4):456–476.

West, C., ed. 1984. *Routine complications: Troubles with talk between doctors and patients.* Bloomington: Indiana University Press.

Witherspoon, G. 1977. *Language and art in the Navajo universe.* Ann Arbor: University of Michigan Press.

Woiche, I. 1992. *Annikadel: The history of the universe as told by the Achumawi Indians of California.* Recorder and ed. Merriam, C. Hart. Tucson: University of Arizona Press.

Young, J. C. 1982. *Medical choice in a Mexican village.* New Brunswick, NJ: Rutgers University Press.

Part II

Interventions in Review

Chapter 6

Knowledge, Attitudes, and Behavior of Alaska Native Women Regarding Cervical and Breast Cancer

Anne P. Lanier and Janet J. Kelly

INTRODUCTION

Cancer is the leading cause of death among Alaska Native women. Between 1984 and 1988 cervical cancer was the fourth most frequently diagnosed invasive cancer in Alaska Native women. Cervical cancer incidence for Alaska Native women in this period was nearly twice that of U.S. whites (Lanier et al. 1996, 750). Prior to 1988, varied and sometimes conflicting cervical cancer prevention guidelines were recommended for U.S. women. However, in 1988 certain national groups agreed on the following recommendation: that all sexually active women, and all women over the age of eighteen years, have an annual Pap smear for three consecutive years and, following three normal Pap tests, follow a less frequent Pap smear schedule as advised by the physician (American College of Obstetricians and Gynecologists 1993, 1). However, the Indian Health Service has consistently recommended that all American Indian and Alaska Native women have annual Pap test starting at age eighteen or when they become sexually active.

Most studies assessing the level of compliance with Pap test recommendations are based on self-reported information. The Behavioral Risk Factor Surveillance System (BRFSS) 1988 and 1989 survey results of over 8,000 black and white women indicate that the proportion of women by state who reported having Pap smears in the last twelve months ranged from 49% to 75% in 1988 and from 54% to 73% in 1989 (Ackermann et al. 1992, 22). A 1987 National Health Interview Survey (NHIS) of 12,000 white, black, Hispanic, and all other race/ethnic groups found that 73% of women reported having had one Pap in the previous three years (Harlan et al. 1991, 887). Further analysis of the NHIS 1987 survey showed that 38% of women interviewed said that they had had a Pap in the last year (Calle et al. 1993, 57). Interviews conducted among Native American women from South Dakota indicated that 60% of the women reported a Pap in the last year

(Minhas 1993). A medical record review of Yaqui Indian women in Arizona for years 1986–1990 showed annual Pap rates ranging from 31 to 36% (Gordon et al. 1994, 99). Data for Alaska Native women showed that in 1991, 83% of women aged eighteen and over (excluding women with hysterectomies) reported having had a Pap test in the last two years (*Healthy Alaskans 2000* 1994, 144). Self-reporting has been shown to overestimate the prevalence of Pap screening in some populations (Sawyer et al. 1989, 1036; Fruchter et al. 1992, 421; McKenna et al. 1992, 288). Data on Pap screening based on medical records for Alaska Native women were not available prior to our project.

The Alaska Native Women's Health Project was one of four American Indian/Alaska Native Avoidable Mortality Projects funded by the National Cancer Institute. The goals of the Alaska project were to determine baseline Pap prevalence among Alaskan Native women, identify barriers to health care services, provide educational materials and counseling on women's health issues, evaluate changes in knowledge and behavior as a result of intervention, and establish a women's clinic based on women's needs and suggestions about cancer and cancer screening services. This chapter describes the results reported by women at their initial interview, associations between reported knowledge and behavior, and changes in knowledge following intervention.

METHODS

Women eligible for the study included Alaska Natives, members of a federally recognized American Indian/Alaska Native group or tribe who were at least twenty years of age (on 1 January 1992), residents of Anchorage, Alaska, and women who made at least one visit to the Alaska Native Medical Center (ANMC) during 1989–1991. (The total number of eligible women registered at ANMC was 5,889). In accordance with treaty agreements, health care is provided to all Alaska Natives at no cost. Nearly 20% of the total Alaska Native population resides in Anchorage, and of them an estimated 90% receive health care at ANMC.

Eligible women were stratified by five-year age groups, and samples were drawn to enroll fifty individuals in each age group. Of the 611 women contacted and to whom the project was explained, a total of 481 (79%) agreed to participate.

All 481 completed a face-to-face, forty-five-minute knowledge, attitude, and behavior survey (KAB 1). The survey instrument included questions developed specifically for Alaska Native women, using questions taken from other surveys, including the Behavioral Risk Factor Survey (BRFSS, Centers for Disease Control). Women were asked about their knowledge of cervical and breast cancer, cancer risk factors, and cancer screening tests (Pap tests, breast examinations, breast self-examination, and mammography), smoking, sexually transmitted diseases (STDs), and their opinions about preventive services provided at ANMC. A second interview (KAB 2) was administered to 200 age-stratified, randomly selected women who had participated in the first interview. In addition to some of the same questions asked in the first interview, the second interview included questions about the intervention and the project's new evening clinic services. Women were given twenty dollars upon completion of each interview to help defray costs of travel, baby-sitters, or loss of work because of their participation.

INTERVENTION

Prior to the initiation of the project, women's health services had been provided only on weekdays during daytime hours, and appointments had been scheduled for twenty minutes in length. There were no appointment reminders, and women were advised of their Pap test results only if abnormal. The project intervention began during and following the first interview. Women were given assistance with scheduling their health maintenance appointments; offered a choice of day or evening clinics; offered advice and educational materials on women's health issues; and were contacted subsequent to their interview to remind them of schedule, or routine appointments to follow-ups of Pap or other test results.

Intervention included educational and motivational materials developed and distributed by the project staff to the participants. The materials included calendars with reminder stickers, a Pap test brochure developed specifically for the target population; and information on other health topics requested by participants at the time of interview. Educational materials were tailored to women's requests and distributed in two mailings. During the course of the project, the staff developed a culturally sensitive educational brochure and video about the importance of cervical cancer screening.

Following the first interview, an evening women's clinic was opened for three nights a week in response to the women's comments and suggestions. Only women (nurses and nurse practitioners) staffed the clinic. Appointments were scheduled for an hour, to provide comprehensive services and allow time to counsel women on any health issues they wished to discuss. The services offered in the evening women's health clinic included physical exam, pap test, breast exam, mammogram appointment, health education (counseling and handouts), tobacco cessation counseling, family planning and birth control, STD and HIV counseling, menopause counseling, nutrition and weight counseling, hormone replacement therapy, immunization update, blood draw and lab tests, pharmacy services, and appointments for specialty clinics.

ANALYSIS

Questions were asked to assess women's knowledge in three categories: breast and cervical cancer prevention and smoking-related health effects. Each question counted as a fraction of the total number of questions for a particular category; for example, cervical cancer category had six questions, each worth one-sixth of a point. The breast cancer section included four questions and the smoking section twelve, respectively. The three categories were worth one point each. We defined a high score as one greater than the mean for questions correctly answered on the first interview. Thus if the mean for questions correctly answered was 3.2, a "high" score was correctly answering four or more questions, while three or fewer correctly answered questions was a "low" score.

As noted, many questions were the same in the first and second interview. Improvement in knowledge following intervention was assessed by comparing the percentages of correct responses to identical questions in the first and second interviews.

We analyzed differences between age groups and differences in answers to knowledge questions before and after intervention. All chi-square and McNemar's tests were performed using Epi Info ver. 6.0 (Dean et al. 1996).

RESULTS

The ethnic distribution of the 481 participants—43% Eskimo, 36% Indian, and 21% Aleut—approximates the distribution of ethnic groups of adult Native women living in Anchorage (42% Eskimo, 41% Indian, 17% Aleut). Table 6.1 shows responses of interviews by ten-year age groups to questions on demographic factors and reproductive history.

Educational level differed by age group. A higher proportion of women age fifty and over did not complete high school. More of the older women were single at the time of the interview, had had three or more pregnancies, and had had a hysterectomy, than was the case for younger women. Younger women more often reported sex initiation before the age of sixteen than did older women. Women of the fifty to fifty-nine age group reported the highest use of female hormones other than for birth control. Women ages twenty to twenty-nine reported the highest use (both current and ever) of birth control pills.

Fourteen percent of participants reported having had cancer (6% cervical, 4% breast, 1% colorectal, and 3% other cancers). Nine percent reported that a mother or sister had been diagnosed with breast cancer. Among all women, 59% had breast-fed.

Twenty-two percent of women had had a hysterectomy. Reasons for hysterectomy included abnormal bleeding (35%), fibroids/benign tumors (26%), cancer (13%), or other reasons (27%).

At the initial interview, women said that their health was either excellent (18%), good (52%), fair (25%), or poor (4%). Among women who completed a second interview, 67% stated that their health status was unchanged since the first interview. Nearly equal numbers of women reported that their health had improved (20%) or become worse (18%) over the study period. Most women (94%) said that they went to the Alaska Native Medical Center when they were sick; 9% said that they had sought a traditional healer for spiritual needs or health care at some time in their lives.

Women were asked what they considered the most serious health problem for Alaska Native women; in the first interview, 53% of women identified alcoholism and 20% cancer. In the second interview, more women named cancer (31%) as the most serious problem, but not above alcoholism (32%).

Women were asked a series of open-ended questions about the preventive services they received at the ANMC clinics. Asked what problems they encountered in getting an appointment at the ANMC women's clinics, some women (29%) said they did not have any problems with scheduling, whereas one-third (33%) said there were insufficient appointment slots and that they had to wait too long for an appointment. When asked what changes they would prefer in available appointments hours, 30% said current hours were satisfactory, 36% said they wanted evening hours, 6% wanted weekend hours for women who work or have children, and 5% wanted more appointment slots made available. Of women asked what problems they had with the clinic staff or quality of care they received at the clinics, half (49%) responded that they did not have any problems with the services, 17% said they had to wait too long in the clinic for the health care provider, 12% remarked that the staff attitudes were poor, 10% said they wanted more patient education and staff-patient communication, and 6% said they wanted more personal care (that is, more attention paid to them). Women said that they preferred a female health care provider for Pap tests (48% in first interview, 64% in the second interview), and some said they would refuse a Pap if only male health care providers were available (18% and 21%, first and second interviews, respectively).

Women were asked if and how they had learned the results of their last Pap test. Half (51%) of the women had been told of the results of their Pap test. Of those informed, 35% said it had been by phone, 34% at a follow-up visit, 25% by mail, and 3% had called the clinic to get the results. Eight percent of the 481 participants in the first interview and 10% of 200 women in the second interview reported that their last Pap had been abnormal. Nearly all women (98%) reported in the second interview that they wanted to know the result of their Pap test (even if normal). They felt that notification by mail (41%), phone (34%), either mail or phone (20%), or at follow-up appointment (5%) was satisfactory.

At the second interview, women were asked if they had received a reminder to get a Pap test. The majority of women (77%) reported receiving a reminder. Ninety-one percent had received a reminder by mail; 58% had received a phone call reminder only, or in addition to a written reminder. Nearly all who received the reminders said they liked them; 96% who received written reminders liked them and 97% who were called appreciated the phone calls. When asked at the end of the first interview if they would like more information on cervical or breast cancer screening, or any other health information, 69% of the women said yes.

Responses to knowedge questions for the sample of 200 women are not statistically different from the responses for the entire study population of 481 women.

Table 6.2 compares correct responses for selected knowledge questions asked on both interviews. Significant improvement was documented on individual questions and summary scores. In the first interview, 55% of the women scored high in knowledge of cervical cancer, correctly answering four or more of six questions. In the second interview, 77% of the women scored high.

On breast cancer questions in the first interview, the majority (70%) of women scored high, correctly answering all four questions. In the second interview only slightly more (77%) scored high.

Knowledge of cancers and illnesses caused by smoking was assessed in twelve smoking questions. Only 37% of the women had high scores (at least eight out of twelve questions correct) in the first interview, whereas in the second interview 71% of women had high scores.

Of all three knowledge categories combined, there was marked improvement; 49% scored high in the first interview and 76% in the second interview.

We compared knowledge with age, education, ethnicity, and marital status. Age was associated with cervical and breast cancer knowledge (high vs. not high) scores in both interviews. Women sixty years of age appeared to be less knowledgeable about cervical and breast cancer and other categories than other age groups. Knowledge of smoking effects did not differ substantially by age. Among women who had not completed high school, knowledge of cervical and breast cancer prevention and smoking hazards was significantly lower than among those who had completed high school, in both interviews. Knowledge scores did not differ by ethnic group or marital status on either interview.

Women who had a personal history of cancer (14% of 481 women) or who had a mother or sister diagnosed with breast cancer (9%) did not score higher in cervical or breast cancer knowledge or knowledge of smoking hazards than women who had never had a diagnosis of breast cancer or had no family member with breast cancer.

Table 6.3 shows that in the first interview, 72% of the women reported that their last Pap test had been within the twelve months prior to the interview. The percentage of women reporting Pap test within the last twelve months differed significantly by age. Women aged sixty years and older reported fewer Pap tests than did younger women. Overall, 44% of women reported doing breast self-exams monthly. Women said that they had learned to do breast self-exams from a health care provider (80%) and/or from written educational material (20%). In the second interview, the eighty-eight women who did not regularly practice breast-self exams were asked to state their reasons. Some women gave multiple answers. More than half of the women (63%) said they did not remember to do breast self-exams, 16% said they have no reason to be concerned about breast cancer, 16% said they did not know how to do a breast self-exam correctly or that they were unale to interpret what they feel, 8% said that they do not like to do breast self-exams, and 3% said they are afraid of what they might find. However, many women who do regular breast self-exams stated that they did know how to do a breast self-exam correctly.

Sixty-nine percent of women reported an annual breast exam by a provider. Reports of annual breast exams were significantly different by age. More women aged fifty to fifty-nine than other age groups reported annual breast exams. Women (n = 38) who reported never having had a breast exam by a health care provider gave as their reasons that they did not know to have one done (27%), were not ill and so did not need one (23%), did not like the exam (7%), or had never asked for an exam (10%). Other reasons included being too busy or inconvenient appoitnment hours.

Of all women interviewed, less than 40% reported having had a mammogram in the twelve months before the first interview. However, among the 170 women aged fifty and over, 67% reported having had a mammogram within the last year, and 82% said they had had a mammogram in the last two years. Five percent of all women reported more than one sex partner in the previous six months; 18% reported having had two or more of seven different types of STDs (gonorrhea, syphilis, venereal warts or HPV, genital herpes, chlamydia, HIV/AIDS and trichomonas). More than half of the women (59%) were correct in their reporting of STD prevention methods. Among women reporting partners, 90% said that their partner helped in the prevention of STDs.

Of all women interviewed, 43% were current smokers. Women between ages twenty and twenty-nine had the highest proportion of smokers (52%).

Women with a history of cancer did not differ from women who never had a diagnosis of cancer with regard to annual breast exams (71% cancer-diagnosed women had annual breast exams vs. 68% cancer-free women) or to reported monthly breast self-exams (51% cancer-diagnosed women had monthly breast self-exams vs. 42% of cancer-free women).

An association was found between knowledge and reported behavior. Women who had high knowledge summary scores were significantly more likely than women with low scores to report that they received annual breast exams by a provider (74% vs. 63%) and to name correct STD prevention methods (65% vs. 52%). They were less likely to report full-term birth before age eighteen (10% vs. 16%) or three or more pregnancies (62% vs. 71%).

DISCUSSION

This study was the first to examine women's health issues, particularly cancer screening issues, among Alaska Natives. Responses on initial interviews suggest that women know more about breast cancer than about cervical cancer, although questions were not necessarily of equal difficulty. All breast cancer questions were correctly answered by 81% or more of the women. Only 61% of women interviewed had heard of a test for "cervical cancer." Less than half of the women said they knew of ways they could reduce their risk of cervical cancer.

Most women understood that smoking contributes to heart disease, cancers of the mouth, throat, larynx, esophagus, and lung and to low-birth-weight infants, but few knew the relationship between smoking and cervical and bladder cancers, prior to participation in the project. More than half of the women said they knew a great deal about HIV/AIDS, yet fewer than one-third said they knew much about any one of six other sexually acquired diseases. These differences in knowledge of health and disease prevention may be a result of national campaigns that have focused on breast cancer, HIV/AIDS, and smoking. Public health messages for the prevention of cervical cancer have not been targeted nationally.

Our sample included approximately equal numbers of women of each five-year age group, and it allowed us to compare knowledge, attitudes, and reported behavior among women of different age groups. Older women had less formal education, lower scores on cancer prevention questions, and reported fewer Pap tests but not fewer breast exams. Younger women may have had more frequent visits to health clinics, because of maternal and child health care needs, than older women and thus received more prevention information. Many older women felt they were too old to have a Pap test done or felt that they no longer needed one because they had had a hysterectomy. The proportion of Native women in this study who had had a hysterectomy more than doubled between women in their forties and women in their sixties, however, Pap test rates did not differ markedly between women with and without hysterectomies. Younger women more often reported behaviors that increase their risk for cervical cancer than older women: sex initiation before age sixteen, more than one sex partner in the prior six months, having had two or more STDs, and current smoking. Single women, young and old, were found to have higher risks overall for cancer than women currently living with a partner.

There was an association between knowledge and reported behavior with respect to cancer screening tests. Despite relatively high knowledge rates, less than the optimum number of women reported annual cancer-screening exams, Pap test (72%), breast exam (69%), and monthly breast self-exam (44%).

Among the most important findings were that women who did not get one screening exam were unlikely to get others, and that those less likely to undergo tests for early detection of cancer were those who appear to be at highest risk, based on reported behaviors. These findings have important implications for provision of preventive services. Every clinic visit should provide an opportunity to update preventive health services, including education and counseling.

From the interviews we learned that women wanted to be better informed about women's health issues. Preferences for screening services included more available appointment times, women providers, appointments reminders by phone or mail, and patient notification of screening test results even if normal. Resources from the Centers for Disease Control Breast and Cervical Cancer Early Detection Program have allowed tribal organizations in Alaska to implement lessons learned from the Women's Health Project.

ACKNOWLEDGMENTS

Funded by the National Cancer Institute, Division of Cancer Prevention and Control, Cooperative Agreement with the Indian Health Service (Grant No. UO1CA52242). Project title: Prevention of Cervical Cancer in Alaska Native Women.

The authors would like to express thanks to additional project personnel: James E. Berner, Lucy Billie, Dodie Matsko, Carol Brandall, Michelle Moran, Margaret Galovin, Barbara Stillwater, Teri Gleason, Nancy Sydnam, Pat Taylor,

Caroline Kuether, Barbara Williams, Regina Kuhnley, Kendall Thomas, and the Aleutian Pribilof Island Association, Inc.

The opinions in this paper are those of the authors and do not necessarily reflect the views of the Indian Health Service.

LITERATURE CITED

Ackermann, Susan P., Robert M Brackbill, Barbara A. Bewerse, Nancy E. Cheal, and Lee M. Sanderson. 1992. Cancer screening behaviors among U.S. women: Breast cancer, 1987–1989, and cervical cancer, 1988–1989. *Centers for Disease Control, Surveillance Summaries* 41(SS-2):17–34.

American College of Obstetricians and Gynecologists. 1993. Cervical cancer cytology: Evaluation and management of abnormalities. *ACOG Technical Bulletin* 183:17.

Calle, Eugenia E., W. Dana Flanders, Michael J. Thun, and Linda M. Martin. 1993. Demographic predictors of mammography and Pap smear screening in U.S. women. *American Journal of Public Health* 83(1):53–60.

Dean, Andrew G., Jeffrey A. Dean, Anthony H. Burton, and Richard C. Dicker. 1996. Epi Info, version 6: A wordprocessing, database, and statistical program for epidemiology on microcomputers. Centers for Disease Control, Atlanta, GA.

Fruchter, Rachel G., Kathie Rones, Tracy Roth, Carolyn A. Webber, Lois Camilien, and John G. Boyce. 1992. Pap smear histories in a medical clinic: Accuracy of patients' self-reports. *New York State Journal of Medicine* 92(10): 421–424.

Gordon, P. R., D. Campos-Outcalt, L. Steele, and C. Gonzales. 1994. Mammography and Pap smear screening of Yaqui Indian women. *Public Health Reports* 109(1):99–103.

Harlan, Linda C., Amy B. Bernstein, and Larry G. Kessler. 1991. Cervical cancer screening: Who is not screened and why? *American Journal of Public Health* 81(7):885–890.

Healthy Alaskans 2000. 1994. Juneau, AK: Department of Health and Social Services, 144–148.

Lanier, Anne P., Janet J. Kelly, Bonnie Smith, Annette P. Harpster, Harvey Tanttia, Claudette Amadon, Dennis Beckworth, Charles Key, and Anna Marie Davidson. 1996. Alaska Native cancer update: Incidence rates 1989–1993. *Cancer Epidemiology, Biomarkers and Prevention* 5:749–751.

McKenna, Matthew T., Marjorie Speers, Katherine Mallin, and Richard Warnecke. 1992. Agreement between patient self-reports and medical records for Pap smear histories. *American Journal of Preventive Medicine* 8(5):287–291.

Minhas, Sumanjit S. 1993. Views held by Native American women concerning Papanicolaou (Pap) screening and uptake of Pap smears within this population. Report to the department of Epidemiology, Public Health Service, Sioux San Hospital, Rapid City, SD.

Sawyer, John A., Jo Anne Earp, Robert Fletcher, Fedora F. Daye, and Tonja M. Wynn. 1989. Accuracy of women's self-report of their last Pap smear. *American Journal of Public Health* 79(8):1036–1037.

Table 6.1
Self-Reported Demographic Factors and Reproductive History of 481 Women's Health Project Participants, by Age

Participants (n=481)	Age 20-29 %	Age 30-39 %	Age 40-49 %	Age 50-59 %	Age 60+ %	All Ages %
Age	20	21	23	19	16	100
Education less than high school graduate*	13	14	16	37	62	26
Marital status = single*	34	32	46	41	65	42
Age at first sex <16*	34	34	16	15	9	22
Age at first full term birth <18	15	12	7	14	17	13
Had >3 pregnancies*	46	66	56	82	90	66
Patient h istory of cancer†	6	8	11	20	31	14
Mother and / or sister had breast cancer	7	12	6	9	10	9
Breastfed children*	53	68	46	59	73	59
Ever used birth control pills*	92	83	77	57	22	69
Currently use birth control pills*	23	10	3	0	1	8
Ever used hormones other than for birth control*	9	13	27	62	42	30
Now use hormones other than for for birth control*	5	3	15	42	23	17
Had hysterectomy*	0	4	25	38	51	22

Notes: * Significant association between age group and response ($p < 0.05$).
† Based on participant report, unconfirmed by medical chart review.

Table 6.2

Comparison of Correct Responses for Select Interview Questions of Knowledge of Cancer Prevention before and after Intervention for 200 Women

Knowledge Category	Question (first and second interviews)	First Interview n = 200 % Correct	Second Interview n = 200 % Correct
Cervical Cancer	Heard of test for cervical cancer	60	72*
	Names test: Pap†	73	73
	Pap if using birth control pills	89	92
	Pap after menopause	85	92*
	Can a woman reduce her risks of cervical cancer	45	79*
	Specific ways to reduce risks☐	81	80
Breast Cancer	See provider for lump	98	100
	All lumps not cancerous	80	84
	Breast self exam once/month	96	99
	Breast exam annually	92	91
Smoking Hazards	Low birth weight infants	79	89*
	Breathing illness	92	99*
	Ear problems	29	54*
	Heart disease	86	92
	Lung cancer	99	99
	Cervical cancer	22	63*
	Skin cancer	14	6*
	Mouth cancer	79	93*
	Throat cancer	91	97*
	Laryngeal cancer	89	96*
	Esophageal cancer	75	92*
	Bladder cancer	15	42*

Table 6.2 (continued)
Comparison of Correct Responses for Selected Interview Questions of Knowledge of Cancer Prevention before and after Intervention for 200 Women

Knowledge Category	Question (first and second interviews)	First Interview n = 200 % Correct	Second Interview n = 200 % Correct
Summary Scores	Cervical cancer high score	55	77*
	Breast cancer high score	70	77
	Smoking hazards high score	37	71*
	All knowledge categories, high score	49	76*

Notes: *First and second interview responses significantly different
   (p < 0.05, McNemar test).
† Of those women who had heard of the test, the percentage who said "Pap" test.
□ Of women who said women can reduce their risks for cervical cancer, the percentage able
   to name correctly a specific way to reduce the risk.

Table 6.3

Cancer Screening and High-Risk Behaviors Reported by Women on First Interview, by Age

Reported Behavior	Age 20-29 %	Age 30-39 %	Age 40-49 %	Age 50-59 %	Age 60+ %	All Ages %
Pap (prior 12 months)	78	76	70	74	58	72
Monthly breast self-exam	33	42	47	52	44	44
Breast exam by provider (prior 12 months)	63	73	61	80	68	69
Mammogram (prior 12 months)	4	18	46	68	66	39
More than 1 sex partner in 6 months	14	3	6	2	0	5
Know STD prevention method(s)	77	71	62	52	25	59
Had two or more types of STDs	26	31	17	10	3	18
Current Smoker	52	42	44	41	35	43

Chapter 7

"Pathways to Health": A School-Based Cancer Prevention Project for Southwestern Native American Youth

Sally M. Davis and Leslie Cunningham-Sabo

The Centers for Disease Control and Prevention have reported that about half of all factors that influence an individual's chances of surviving to age sixty-five relate to lifestyle behaviors. Approximately 30% of all cancer deaths correspond to tobacco use (*Cancer Control* 1986). Numerous research articles link specific foods or nutrients to certain types of cancer (Wynder and Gori 1977), and about 50% of cancer incidence is related to diet (Committee on Diet and Health et al. 1989). Lifestyle behavioral goals of both the National Cancer Institute and the American Cancer Society include avoidance of all tobacco products, decreased consumption of dietary fat (to less than 30% of daily calories), and increased consumption of dietary fiber (to 20–30 grams per day) (Butrum et al. 1988; Nixon 1990).

In the past, strong cultural traditions and rural isolation protected many Southwestern Native American peoples from certain risk factors associated with cancer, such as commercial tobacco use and high-fat foods. However, this protective isolation is disappearing. With its loss, new patterns of morbidity and mortality, associated in part with the adoption of Western lifestyles, have surfaced (Welty 1991). This alteration of lifestyle will likely lead to an increasing presence of cancer risk factors and disease among Southwestern American Indians.

The lung cancer mortality rate among native groups living in Arizona and New Mexico remains consistently lower than that of other U.S. tribes (Valway 1991, 113). Environmental and cultural factors—for instance, limited smoking—undoubtedly play a role in this difference. Previous research (Harris and Ford 1988), however, indicates that tobacco use among young American Indians in the Southwest may be increasing. As acculturation of Southwestern Indians rises, tobacco-related diseases may correspondingly increase (U.S. Department of Health and Human Services 1986).

Current rates of diet-related cancers among American Indians remain generally lower than those of the U.S. population as a whole (Indian Health Service 1990). However, recent trends towards higher-fat, lower-fiber diets among some Native American populations suggest that their risk for these types of cancer may increase, as have observed prevalence patterns for diabetes and cardiovascular disease. Like children elsewhere in the United States (Kimm et al. 1990), Native American children derive approximately 35% of their daily calories from fat (Sugarman, White, and Gilbert 1990).

Schools, perhaps more than any other single agency in society, can help young people develop healthful lifestyle behaviors (Allensworth and Kolbe 1987). Such behaviors can improve school performance, reduce dropout rates, and better students' health in adulthood. Cultural beliefs and practices exert strong influences on decisions made in daily living, including choices related to personal health (Jackson and Broussard 1987). For native people, as for all people, desired health behavior must be modeled and demonstrated within a cultural context if favorable lifestyle changes are to be brought about (Hughes and Aluli 1991).

In response to a growing concern of community members, a group of school employees, health care providers, University of New Mexico Prevention Research Center investigators, and health educators developed, implemented, and evaluated a prevention model known as "Pathways to Health" specifically for American Indian children and their families. The model features a health-promotion curriculum discouraging tobacco use and encouraging a low-fat and high-fiber diet; it includes a social influences component, intergenerational activities, and storytelling; a family component; and school staff training and development. (For a more complete description of the program, refer to previous publications by these authors: Cunningham-Sabo and Davis 1993; Davis et al. 1995; Cunningham-Sabo et al. 1996; Davis, Cunningham-Sabo, and Lambert 1999.)

POPULATION

From fall 1992 to spring 1995, the Pathways to Health project was implemented in twelve American Indian schools in the rural Southwest. The schools were either public, tribal, or operated by the Bureau of Indian Affairs (BIA). Two additional schools participated only in pilot test activities, in spring 1992. All the schools were in rural areas; some were extremely isolated, while others were closer to manufactured goods and services. Many of the schools and the communities in which they were located were in designated rural or "frontier" areas, with six or fewer persons per square mile: they were fifty to 200 miles from a major metropolitan center. People who lived closer to the metropolitan area or other "towns" were considered to have access to grocery stores and other markets.

The intervention included fifth and seventh-grade students, since children this age possess many of the basic skills needed to participate competently in an interactive curriculum and encounter peer pressure and other social influences. They represent two developmental ages.

A total of 1589 students participated in the project in the three school years between fall 1992 and spring 1995. Ethnically the students consisted predominantly of American Indians (95.8%), fairly evenly divided by gender (51.9% boys and 48.1% girls) and by grade (51.2% fifth graders and 48.7% seventh graders).

RESEARCH DESIGN

The research was quasi-experimental pretest-posttest, with schools randomly assigned to one of three conditions: curriculum only; curriculum plus family component; or control (delayed intervention). The curriculum-plus-family component was added to randomly assigned schools in the fourth year of funding (third year in the school). The delayed-intervention schools received an alternative health education curriculum initially and the Pathways to Health curriculum in the final (fifth) year of the project.

METHODS

In order to collect descriptive baseline data and determine the effectiveness of the health promotion curriculum, Pathways to Health staff developed, pilot tested, and further refined pre- and posttest instruments to assess students' knowledge, attitudes, and self-reported behaviors related to the curriculum themes. Staff administered these instruments following the project's standardized procedures, before and after the implementation of the curriculum (approximately seven months apart). The project used chi-square tests to evaluate curriculum effects for discrete variables for each grade, with the alpha level set at .05 for all analyses. Future analyses will further evaluate program results.

CURRICULUM

During the two-year curriculum-development process, the multicultural and multidisciplinary project team convened separate focus groups of American Indian teachers, parents, and school administrators to identify key concepts and appropriate methods for school-based implementation and to assure reliability and sensitivity to cultural values. Drawing from the rich cultural heritage of beliefs, values, and customs of the participants, the team identified the following cultural concepts and used them to design the curriculum: learning through observation and practice (Johns-Steiner 1975); learning from storytelling (Johns-Steiner 1975); learning metaphorically (Havinghurst et al. 1946; More 1987); holistic learning (Rhodes 1994); learning by trial and error (Little Soldier 1992); learning cooperatively (Swisher and Deyhe 1989); and learning through reflection (Gilliland 1992).

The Pathways to Health curriculum incorporates these cultural concepts into a sixteen-lesson educational program that uses experiential activities and presents concepts through storytelling. Using the "Coyote" trickster character, a metaphor for social influences, as the central motif of the curriculum, it teaches children ways to avoid negative social pressures and improve their health decision-making skills. Coyote is a well known figure for a number of American Indian tribes, and there are many stories telling how he uses his cleverness to trick other animals into satisfying his greed. His stunts usually backfire, with Coyote becoming the butt of his own jokes.

As in models developed for and used with the Checkerboard Cardiovascular Curriculum (Harris et al. 1988) and the Southwest Cardiovascular Curriculum (Davis et al. 1995, 26)—two earlier projects developed for fifth-grade students in similar populations— intergenerational activities are an important part of the curriculum. Elders from the local communities are included as teachers in the curriculum to teach the children about traditional Native American ways that recognize the importance of preventing illness and promoting a healthful lifestyle. These presentations by the elders do not imply that it would be best to return to "the old ways" but rather integrate historically valuable information into the lessons so as to validate the culture of the students (Davis 1994). Students also interview their parents and grandparents about "the old ways," by which they grew much of the food they ate, were more physically active, and restricted tobacco for sacred uses.

Written materials as well as a videotape, *Life in Balance*, were developed to enhance the curriculum and the family activities. In *Life in Balance*, six American Indian adults who serve as role models describe their personal journeys to a more healthful balance in their lives through improved behaviors. In addition, the curriculum development team took extreme care in creating curriculum materials, such as the easy-to-use teacher guide, student workbook, and family components, to make them culturally and scientifically relevant and appropriate. The team designed the family materials with a low-literacy audience in mind as well, using some of the techniques described by Doak et. al (1985).

Social Learning Theory (SLT) (Perry et al. 1990) provided the theoretical base for the Pathways to Health curriculum, which emphasizes two primary behavioral goals: selecting and preparing a diet low in fat and high in fiber, fruits, and vegetables; and avoiding cigarettes and smokeless tobacco products. The curriculum uses constructs from SLT to promote changes in the children's environment supporting them in developing healthy behaviors. The lessons highlight positive role models and provide opportunities to practice resisting pressures to use tobacco. For example, students write anti-tobacco skits and then perform them for their classmates. Role plays and group activities provide practice and social support for selecting lower-fat foods and refusing to smoke cigarettes or chew tobacco. The curriculum also expands children's skills and experience in reading food labels and making healthful choices. Students are asked to bring packaged food nutrition labels to class to review with their teacher and classmates.

TEACHER TRAINING AND SUPPORT

The project team included school staff members in all aspects of the Pathways to Health program, in order to enhance its acceptance in the schools and to promote its continuance after the project funding ended. As a crucial part of this inclusion, teachers attended a two-day Educators' Training session at the University of New Mexico prior to teaching the curriculum. Their training, for which they could enroll for university credit, included the program rationale and the content and teaching methods of the curriculum. Sample lessons were modeled, and elders from participating communities demonstrated the intergenerational lesson activity. The training sessions also offered intercultural communication workshops and addressed other topics related to culture and health promotion considerations.

After teachers had finished teaching the curriculum, a project staff member completed a one-on-one face-to-face process evaluation interview with them. The purpose was to determine the teachers' and students' reactions to the curriculum and, where appropriate, the family component. While the comments from teachers varied widely, several themes emerged: the students had really enjoyed the hands-on nature of the curriculum; they had enjoyed tasting new foods; and the teachers had found the use of the sponge "lungs" to demonstrate the effect of tobacco smoke on lungs, and the graphic pictures of diseased oral tissue due to chewing tobacco, quite effective. The teachers also appreciated the cultural relevance of the curriculum. Comments on the intergenerational activities were consistently positive.

FAMILY COMPONENT

The family-based companion component to the Pathways to Health classroom curriculum began in June 1993. Project staff held focus groups with parents to identify appropriate program implementation strategies; subsequently, the project team developed lessons and activities based on family input. In fall 1994, the five-week curriculum began with a kickoff party at the participating schools, followed by three weeks of take-home activity packets for the students to complete with family members. The culminating activity, a wrap-up party—again held at school—invited students and family members to celebrate the program.

In general, participation rates for the kickoff party, wrap-up party, and take-home assignments were higher than had been anticipated by teachers. Kickoff party attendance rates ranged from 27% of students in one school to 86% in another. The completion rate of take-home assignments ranged from 27% in one seventh-grade class to 69% in one fifth-grade class. In general, a higher percentage of students completed these worksheets if the teacher was actively involved and reminded them of this homework.

RESULTS

Currently little data exists on the health knowledge, attitudes, and behaviors of American Indian children and youth. The data presented here are important contributions to that small body of information.

Pretest data indicated that students' favorite foods were pizza, hamburgers, and tacos. Only 35% of students reported consuming two or more daily servings of fruit, which is the U.S. Dietary Guidelines recommendation, and only 19.3% reported more than once-a-day intake of vegetables (see also Teufel, this volume). The mean score (percent correct responses) for questions on common food sources of dietary fat and fiber and other cancer-related nutrition knowledge questions was 45.2% and 57.9% for fifth and seventh grade students, respectively.

Other selected pretest results have been previously published (Davis et al. 1995; Cunningham-Sabo et al. 1996), but the following summary, comparing students' pre- and posttest responses on tobacco questions, represents the most complete report to date of the data obtained on the project.

SMOKELESS TOBACCO BEHAVIOR CHANGES

Students were asked questions related to current use of tobacco, potential future use, and likelihood of use if offered by a best friend. Approximately 92% of both fifth-grade intervention and control students were not current users of smokeless tobacco at either pre- or posttest, and nearly 65% of both groups indicated they would not use tobacco even if their best friend offered it to them. Fifty-three percent of both groups were sure they would never use smokeless tobacco. No differences were found in the proportions of the responses between intervention and control groups of fifth graders for any of the five questions.

The seventh-grade students' self-reports of smokeless tobacco use present a different picture, however. Among those who were not current users at pretest, almost 92% of the intervention students remained nonusers at posttest, compared with 82% in the control group, and approximately 5% of the intervention nonusers became users by posttest, compared with more than 9% in the control group.

There was a difference between seventh-grade intervention and control students in their responses to the question about expected use if a best friend offered them smokeless tobacco, with 43% of students in the control group and 58% of the intervention group answering they would not accept. More of the students in the control group remained unsure (16% of control vs. 10% of intervention students) about what they would do if offered smokeless tobacco by their best friend.

Overall, few seventh-grade students in either group consistently thought that they would ever use smokeless tobacco, but more of the control students continued to think they would use it, or were unsure, at posttest. Nearly half (48%) of the intervention students remained sure they would never use smokeless tobacco, compared with 38% in the control group. Overall, students in the intervention groups reported that they were less likely to use smokeless tobacco in the future.

SMOKING TOBACCO BEHAVIOR CHANGES

No differences in pre- and posttest change categories occurred among fifth graders' self-reports for the five survey questions. More than three-fourths of the students in both intervention and control groups reported not smoking at both pre- and posttest, and more than 85% indicated they had not smoked within twenty-four hours of either test.

Among seventh graders, several differences appeared in pre- and posttest change categories regarding recent smoking behavior and likelihood of smoking in the future, and unfortunately these differences were in an unexpected direction. The intervention students were more likely to have reported they had smoked within twenty-four hours of each test and were more likely to have smoked before the posttest when they had not smoked before the pretest. In addition, the intervention group was more likely to think they will smoke cigarettes eventually, with nearly 25% answering "yes" both pre- and posttest, and 15% changing from "unsure" on the pretest to "yes" on the posttest.

Overall, based on preliminary analysis of the data, there was no significant difference in pre- and post-response categories between intervention and control groups in either grade when change in smoking behavior was examined—those who smoked less, the same, or more at posttest compared to pretest.

In general, the participants in this study have low rates of current use of smokeless tobacco, with less than 7% of fifth-grade intervention and control students reporting current use at posttest. Approximately 8% of seventh-grade intervention students reported current use of smokeless tobacco at posttest, and 15% of seventh-grade control students used smokeless tobacco at posttest. Current cigarette use was approximately twice that of smokeless tobacco use in the fifth graders (approximately 14% in both groups at posttest), and the seventh-grade control group reported greater cigarette than smokeless tobacco use (at 25%). Of concern, seventh-grade intervention students reported higher levels of cigarette use (38% "regular" or "sometimes" use at posttest).

DISCUSSION

The difference in reported tobacco behaviors between fifth and seventh-grade students suggest that sixth grade may be a critical transition period for these children. Future health education efforts could be extremely useful in reducing behavioral intentions to take up tobacco use if intensively focused on this grade. Tobacco may also be viewed as more daring or risky during early adolescence, when risk-taking, experimentation, and social acceptance are so important.

Future analyses will explore potential gender and age differences in reported tobacco use and in tobacco knowledge changes. Statistical analyses of the comparison of student pre- and posttest results between curriculum-only schools and curriculum-plus-family schools are also in progress.

SUMMARY AND RECOMMENDATIONS

The Pathways to Health program was very positively received by the communities and schools in which it was tested and implemented. The families that participated in the family component were extremely positive in their comments as well. The need for continued cancer prevention efforts is apparent and has been identified by Southwest tribes as a priority (Osborn et al. 1996). Future cancer prevention and health promotion efforts in general should extend even further beyond the school, to incorporate the extended family and the community.

Another recommendation relates to the importance of implementing prevention programs early. Children are initiated into tobacco use early and need clear no-use messages, skills for resisting negative social influences, and support in not using tobacco. Eating habits also form early; children should be given opportunities to taste nutritious low-fat and high-fiber foods, and to develop skills for making healthy choices. Finally, prevention programs need to continue into middle school to provide social support and more complex skills development for growing up healthy.

LITERATURE CITED

Allensworth, D. D., and L. J. Kolbe. 1987. The comprehensive school health program: Exploring an expanded concept. *Journal of School Health* 57(10):409–12.

Butrum, R. R., C. K. Clifford, and E. Lanza. 1988. NCI dietary guidelines: Rationale. *American Journal of Clinical Nutrition* 48(3 Suppl):888–895.*Cancer control: Objectives for the nation: 1985–2000*. 1986. Division of Cancer Prevention and Control. National Cancer Institute. *NCI Monograph* (2):1–93.

Committee on Diet and Health, Food and Nutrition Board, Commission on Life Sciences, and National Research Council. 1989. Diet and health: Implications for reducing chronic disease risk. Washington, DC: National Academy.

Cunningham-Sabo, L., and S. M. Davis. 1993. Pathways to health: A health promotion and cancer prevention project for American Indian youth. *Alaska Medicine* 35(4):275–278, 296.

Cunningham-Sabo, L. D., S. M. Davis, K. M. Koehler, M. L. Fugate, J. A. DiTucci, and B. J. Skipper. 1996. Food preferences, practices, and cancer-related food and nutrition knowledge of southwestern American Indian youth. *Cancer* 78(7 Suppl):1617–1622.

Davis, S. M. 1994. General guidelines for an effective and culturally sensitive approach to health education. In *The Multicultural Challenge in Health Education*, ed. A. C. Matiella, 117–132. Santa Cruz, CA: ETR Associates.

Davis, S. M., L. Cunningham-Sabo, and L. Lambert. 1999. Pathways to Health: A cancer prevention project for Native American schoolchildren and their families. In *Native outreach: A report to American Indian, Alaska Native and Native Hawaiian communities*, ed. C. Glover and F. Hodge, 75–92. Bethesda, MD: National Cancer Institute.

Davis, S. M., L. C. Lambert, L. Cunningham-Sabo, and B. J. Skipper. 1995. Tobacco use: Baseline results from pathways to health, a school-based project for southwestern American Indian youth. *Preventive Medicine* 24(5):454–460.

Davis, S. M., L. C. Lambert, Y. Gomez, and B. Skipper. 1995. Southwest cardiovascular curriculum project: Study findings for American Indian elementary students. *Journal of Health Education* 26(2 Suppl): S72–81.

Doak, C. C., L. G. Doak, and J. H. Root. 1985. *Teaching patients with low literacy skills*. Philadelphia: J. B. Lippincott.

Gilliland, H. 1992. *Teaching the Native American*. Dubuque, IA: Kendall/Hunt Publishing.

Harris, M. B., S. M. Davis, V. L. Ford, and H. Tso. 1988. The checkerboard cardiovascular curriculum: A culturally oriented program. *Journal of School Health* 58(3):104–107.

Harris, M. B., and V. L. Ford. 1988. Tobacco use in a fifth-grade southwestern sample. *Journal of Early Adolescence* 8(1):83–96.

Havinghurst, R. J., M. K. Gunther, and I. E. Pratt. 1946. Environment and draw-a-man tests: The performance of Indian children. *Journal of Abnormal Social Psychology* 41:50–63.

Hughes, C. K., and N. E. Aluli. 1991. A culturally sensitive approach to health education for Native Hawaiians. *Journal of Health Education* 22(6):387–390. Indian Health Service. 1990. *Regional differences in Indian health*. Rockville, MD: U.S. Public Health Service.

Jackson, M. Y., and B. A. Broussard. 1987. Cultural challenges in nutrition education among American Indians. *Diabetes Educator* 13(1):47–50.

Johns-Steiner, V. 1975. Learning styles among Pueblo children: Final report. Report to National Institute of Education, U.S. Department of Health, Education, and Welfare. University of New Mexico, College of Education.

Kimm, S. Y., P. J. Gergen, M. Malloy, C. Dresser, and M. Carroll. 1990. Dietary patterns of U.S. children: Implications for disease prevention. *Preventive Medicine* 19(4):432–42.

Little Soldier, L. 1992. Working with Native American children. *Young Children* September:15–21.

More, A. J. 1987. Native Indian learning styles: A review for researchers and teachers. *Journal of American Indian Education* 26:17–29.

Nixon, D. W. 1990. Nutrition and cancer: American Cancer Society guidelines, programs, and initiatives. *Ca: Cancer Journal for Clinicians* 40(2):71–75.

Osborn, K. L., S. M. Davis, M. Slattery, A. Giuliano, N. I. Teufel, J. Joe, and C. Ritenbaugh. 1996. Four Corners Research Consortium for Native Americans and cancer research. *Cancer* 78(7 Suppl):1629–1632.

Perry, C. L., T. Baranowski, and G. Parcel. 1990. How individuals, environments, and health behavior interact: Social learning theory. In *Health Behavior and Health Education*, ed. K. Glantz, F. M. Lewis, and B. Fimer, 161–186. San Francisco: Jossey-Bass.

Rhodes, R. W. 1994. *Nuturing learning in Native American students*. Hoteville, AZ: Sonwai.

Sugarman, J. R., L. L. White, and T. J. Gilbert. 1990. Evidence for a secular change in obesity, height, and weight among Navajo Indian schoolchildren. *American Journal of Clinical Nutrition* 52(6):960–966.

Swisher, K., and D. Deyhe. 1989. The styles of learning are different, but the teaching is just the same: Suggestions for teachers of American Indian youth. *Journal of American Indian Education* 28(3):28–32.

U.S. Department of Health and Human Services. 1986. Report of the Secretary's Task Force on Black and Minority Health, executive summary 1. Washington, DC: U.S. Government Printing Office.

Valway, S. E. 1991. *Cancer mortality among Native Americans in the United States: Regional differences in Indian health, 1984–1988 and trends over time, 1968–1987*, 113. Rockville, MD: U.S. Department of Health and Human Services, Public Health Service, Indian Health Service.

Welty, T. K. 1991. Health implications of obesity in American Indians and Alaska Natives. *American Journal of Clinical Nutrition* 53(6 Suppl):1616S–1620S.

Wynder, E. L., and G. B. Gori. 1977. Contribution of the environment to cancer incidence: An epidemiologic exercise. *Journal of National Cancer Institute* 58(4):825–32.

Chapter 8

Smoking Cessation Training and Effectiveness Among African Americans

Bruce Allen, Jr.

BACKGROUND

Smoking now accounts for, or is implicated in, about 30% of all cancer deaths in the United States; it is especially implicated in cancers of the lung, mouth, pharynx, esophagus, pancreas, kidney, and bladder. Studies also suggest an association between smoking and cancer of the cervix (NCI 1998). African Americans die disproportionately more from smoking-related cancers (especially lung cancer) than do most any other population group in America (American Cancer Society 1983, see Miller et al. 1996; Wingo et al. 1998). Recent figures on smoking among African-American adults indicate that this situation will not change in the near future (USDHHS 1994). Smoking prevalence is higher in African-American males than any other group; they make more attempts to quit smoking but are less successful in them than their white counterparts (Burns and Pierce 1992). Consequently, the problem of smoking and cancer is likely to persist for a considerable time.

Physicians are viewed by lay people in general as legitimate sources of information about health promotion and disease prevention. In fact, over 75% of smokers report that they would try to quit smoking if their physician advised them to do so (Brink et al. 1994). However, many physicians do not counsel their patients to quit smoking, because of lack of confidence in their ability to do so or underestimation of their impact (Manley et al. 1992; Gilpin et al. 1993; Brink et al. 1994). Physicians tend to give advice about smoking cessation as treatment for smoking-related health problems rather than as prevention of future diseases. Even in circumstances in which physicians are given a specific algorithm, they are unlikely to follow suggested regimens (Ockene et al. 1994).

Several studies (Glynn et al. 1990; Ockene et al. 1990, 1991, 1994; Kottke et al. 1992; Gilpin et al. 1993; Brink 1994 et al.) have evaluated physician effectiveness in smoking cessation in a wide variety of situations. While it appears that physicians are more effective agents of change with their patients who have a smoking-related disease, those caring for patients without those conditions also have an impact. In a meta-analysis of thirty-nine controlled trials of cessation interventions in medical practice settings (Kottke et al. 1988), researchers found that program success twelve months after the initiation of the intervention was related to: (1) the type of intervention session (group and individual sessions combined were better than either alone); (2) intervention modalities; and (3) the number of reinforcing sessions (see also Ockene et al. 1990, 1991, 1994; Kottke et al. 1992).

OPINIONS, ATTITUDES AND COUNSELING PRACTICES

An extensive search of the literature revealed a scarcity of information regarding intervention trials specifically urging African Americans to quit smoking. A onetime physician-delivered cessation message was given to young African-American women in three Baltimore public family planning clinics (Li et al. 1984) resulting in self-reported long-term cessation rates ranging from 3.1% to 9.9%, with the higher rates found in groups receiving a structured, physician-delivered message. In a more recent study of smoking-cessation counseling among African-American physicians, ninety-six respondents completed a survey of their knowledge, attitudes, and practices (Berman et al. 1997). The race/ethnicity of patients that they served in their practice was mixed, with the majority being African American. These physicians estimated that 30% of their patients were current smokers but that few of them sought cessation counseling. Nearly half (46.8%) of the physicians believed that it is possible to provide effective counseling in a few minutes, but a third of them felt that setting up and maintaining an office protocol for smoking cessation would require a great deal of effort. Explaining smoking-related health risks (71.9%) and enrolling patients in smoking-cessation programs (66.6%) were considered key elements.

Given this general lack of information about African-American smoking cessation patterns and the enormity of the problem of tobacco use among adult African Americans, a six-week pilot study was conducted at a large, urban, public general hospital in 1987 to test the effectiveness of smoking cessation counseling by physicians in training (residents). Adult African-American male and female outpatients were targeted to receive a doctor's message on smoking cessation.

A two-hour training session was developed to provide physicians with information about both well-known health effects of smoking as well as several less-known consequences, such as periodontal disease and premature wrinkling of the skin; the benefits of quitting; ways of dealing with withdrawal; precautions about relapse; and procedures for making individual assessments of patients. During training, didactic presentations were used, as were videotapes of counseling sessions and rehearsals of the procedures by the participants. Among other lessons, trainers talked to residents about the consequences of tobacco use by African Americans as compared to other ethnic and racial groups. Gift certificates, lotteries, and newsletters were distributed to reinforce and help maintain the physicians' motivation.

The major elements in the physician-delivered message were: expressing concern about cigarette smoking and the patient's health, soliciting a commitment to quit smoking by setting a target date to quit "cold turkey" or at least thinking about quitting, and giving patients a pamphlet on quitting smoking. The physicians were told to modify the message to suit their own style of communication and the individual patients' needs. Physicians in the treatment group were instructed to begin counseling at the initial clinic visit and provide reinforcement at subsequent visits.

Ninety-two of the trained physicians counseled from one to eighteen patients identified as smokers by markings on their medical charts. A patient entered the intervention or control group according to which group the doctor was assigned. After obtaining informed consent of the patient, research assistants administered a questionnaire on smoking and a breath test. The patient then met with his or her physician. Research assistants conducted exit interviews after the doctor-patient encounters. The research assistants, who were college students or recent college graduates, all had training in smoking cessation similar to that of the doctors.

The results of exit interviews with patients in both groups revealed that physicians had adhered to the protocol requirements with reasonable consistency. Nearly 70% in the intervention group reported that their doctors either somewhat strongly or very strongly urged them to quit smoking, with only 16% of the control group reporting such advice. Ninety-nine percent of the physicians in the intervention group reported that they had sometimes or often discussed the risks of smoking with their patients who smoked but only 75% had recommended alternatives to smoking and only 32% had given pamphlets or other educational materials to their patients who smoked.

RESULTS

A pilot study was conducted to test the feasibility of procedures, psychometric properties of the instruments, and response rates with smokers from the Internal Medicine and Family Medicine Clinics. One hundred thirty-nine eligible patients were identified during the six-week recruitment period; only eight (5.8%) refused to participate in the study. In contrast to the larger number of physicians assigned to the treatment group, there were seventy-two patients in the control condition and fifty-nine in the treatment group. Data entry and analysis packages were tested; the data-entry error rate was only 0.2%. Statistical analysis of the smoking history and sociodemographic characteristics of the two groups revealed that the groups were indeed similar. Over 85% of the treatment participants indicated that the physician had discussed health risks of smoking and methods of cessation. A similar proportion reported receiving self-help guides, and over half had set a quit date.

THE STUDY

Our baseline data suggested that physicians could integrate a three-to-five minute effective smoking-cessation intervention into routine delivery of care. A five-and-a-half-year study (1987–1992) was designed to assess the impact of smoking-cessation communications upon African-American clients. The setting for this study was the Martin Luther King, Jr./Charles R. Drew Medical Center in Los Angeles, California. The hospital is owned by the county of Los Angeles and operated via an affiliation agreement with the private, nonprofit Charles R. Drew University of Medicine and Science. The facility primarily serves individuals who require publicly financed health services. Patients from the Family Medicine and Internal Medicine Clinics were later supplemented by otorhinolaryngology (ENT) and General Surgery patients, to bolster recruitment.

Study Design

A randomized design was used, with blocking on type of clinic and year of residency of the participating physicians. The physicians in training who had participated in the pilot study took part in the main project. With each new class of physicians in training, a sample constituency was randomly assigned to fill the gaps left by graduating residents. Since there were only four clinics and it was not possible to assess their equivalence in terms of populations, diseases treated, etc., randomization of clinics was deemed inappropriate. For Family and Internal Medicine, random assignment of individual patients within the clinic was considered administratively unfeasible. Consequently, in these clinics individual physicians were either trained or not trained in the intervention. However, it was not possible randomly to assign physicians in ENT and General Surgery, because physicians were not routinely scheduled to attend outpatient clinics. Thus, random assignment of patients was adopted.

On a first visit, a patient entered the study and became a member of the intervention or control group, in accordance with the doctor's status. That patient might return to the clinic and see a different doctor; however, the patient always met with a physician who was assigned to the group designated on the first visit. For instance, if Jake had been placed in the control group, his doctor would be reminded not to counsel him according to protocol used for the intervention group patients. The total estimated sample size of patients (474 patients per group) was based on smoking-cessation rates for the control and treatment groups of 5% and 10% respectively, with $\alpha = .05$, and $\beta = .20$. From the pilot study information, it was expected that a period of eighteen months would be necessary to reach this sample size. In actuality, 515 people made up the intervention group; an additional 571 individuals formed the control group.

Procedures

Patients in the control group (n = 571) continued to receive the usual medical care, and they were followed at the same points in time as those in the intervention group. At entry, patients in the treatment group were asked to complete a baseline questionnaire about smoking and had carbon monoxide (CO) levels assessed. This was followed by a three-to-five-minute counseling session by the physician, focusing on the smoker's own symptoms and health risks, advising cessation, and establishing a target quit date. A patient-physician agreement was signed, and patients were given a self-help pamphlet reinforcing the physician's message, which had been designed by the study group.[1] Postcards were given to the patient to be mailed back at specified intervals to report on progress. A list of community cessation programs was provided to each patient along with information on costs and schedules. The carbon monoxide test and personalized message were repeated at all subsequent visits.

Physicians in the treatment group were notified if their patient was a smoker. A summary sheet of the patient's smoking history was placed on the outside of the patient's medical record. Control group physicians in Family and Internal Medicine received no smoking-cessation training or materials, though it is possible that these physicians offered smoking cessation to patients. Those trained were advised not to share any information about smoking cessation with doctors in the control group. In General Surgery and ENT, where all physicians were trained, prompts were provided as to whether a given patient should be counseled. Exit interviews with patient participants served collected information on whether cessation counseling had occurred and whether a target date for quitting had been set. Inquiries asked, did the doctor talk about the patient's smoking habit? Did the doctor make any suggestions about ways to cease smoking? These interviews occurred after the doctor had left the area.

Follow-up telephone interviews in the intervention and control groups occurred three and twelve months after enrollment to assess current smoking behavior. Every effort was made to minimize losses in follow-up by obtaining three contact names, addresses, and telephone numbers, and searching hospital records. Initial attempts to use other methods, such as mail contact prior to telephone follow-up and tracking through the Postal Service, Department of Motor Vehicles, voter registration records, or property tax records, proved unsuccessful and were not pursued.

Because deception rates among smokers participating in cessation studies are generally high (Ohlin et al. 1976), a biochemical measure was used to validate self-reports of abstinence. Jarvis et al. (1987) showed that cotinine measurements in plasma, saliva, and urine are the best indicators of smoking, with high sensitivity and specificity rates. Thus, salivary cotinine samples were collected by research assistants, at homes or in the clinic, from treatment and control subjects who reported not smoking at three months or twelve months postenrollment. The two saliva samples were used to measure the short and long-term effectiveness of the intervention. Samples were analyzed at the American Health Foundation's laboratory in Valhalla, New York. Expired carbon monoxide measurements were taken on all intervention subjects at initial and return clinic visits.

Letters of congratulations were mailed to the patient and physician when smoking cessation was confirmed. The postcard and congratulatory letters were intended to reinforce physician counseling and prevent relapse.

Other Measures

As in the pilot study, a smoker questionnaire was administered to all consenting patients. It addressed demographic characteristics, smoking history and current behavior, smoking knowledge, strength of intention to quit, probability of success, and environmental cues and supports for smoking cessation. A research assistant administered the questionnaire, answered questions, and filled out the records that were kept on each patient. After the office visit, an exit interview was conducted with participants in the intervention group. The interview measured intention to quit, probability of becoming a nonsmoker within the next three months, and a brief checklist indicating knowledge of intervention content. The postexam checklist was used to monitor physician compliance with the protocol. A modified version also was administered to control subjects to determine if they had been exposed to smoking-cessation information.

Analysis

Data entry and editing were conducted using dBase©, SAS©, and BMDP©. In order to assess the effectiveness of the intervention, logistic regression was used to analyze abstinence; analysis of variance or covariance provided values for amount smoked at follow-up and for abstinence. Both self-reported and biochemically validated abstinence were analyzed as a dependent variables. Potential confounders examined were: quitting history, presence of other smokers in the household, amount smoked, intention to quit, and number of contacts with physician during the study. When outcome information was missing due to refusals or losses to follow up, we followed the intention-to-treat principle in the analysis; we also conducted an analysis that included only individuals with complete information. Constant monitoring of process measures (such as patient accrual rate, exit interviews, and postexam checklist) helped to ensure delivery of key intervention components and maximum adherence to protocols by physicians. Potential contamination resulting from the patient, physician, and study environment was monitored through questionnaires.

RESULTS AND PROCESS EVALUATION

Physician Participants

Implementation of the main study began in 1989 in the Departments of Family Medicine and Internal Medicine. In May 1990 the Department of Otorhinolaryngology (ENT) joined, and in March 1991 General Surgery was added to facilitate participant accrual. A total of 158 physicians in training were eligible and consented to participate in the study.

Patient Participants

One thousand eighty six patients enrolled in the study during a twenty-six-month recruitment period. We had hoped to complete recruitment in eighteen months, but we had overestimated the number of smokers that used this health facility. More than 83% of the 1,304 patients who were eligible agreed to participate. The average quarterly recruitment rate was approximately 121 patients. It should be noted that almost half of the patients were recruited in the Internal Medicine clinic.

In all four departments, the number of males exceeded the number of females; the intervention group was 55.0% male, and the control group was 57.3%. Mean age for both groups was virtually identical (43.6 for the intervention group and 43.5 for the controls). Members of both groups had been on average eighteen years old when they started smoking regularly, had smoked fourteen cigarettes per day, and had been smoking for over twenty-five years. Approximately half of both groups reported smoking their first cigarette within fifteen minutes of waking up, and at least three-quarters smoked again within an hour, indicating a high level of nicotine dependency. Nearly 90% had tried to quit smoking for various lengths of time; again the groups were similar with regard to these variables.

OUTCOME EVALUATION

A total of 960 patients (457 intervention, 503 control) were eligible for three-month interviews, and 756 patients (369 intervention, 387 control) were eligible for twelve-month interviews. Because of protocol violations, 126 patients enrolled during weeks twenty-four through thirty-eight inclusive were not evaluated at three months. A sizeable percentage of participants (37.8%, n = 363) eligible for three-month interviews were lost to follow-up, because of either missing or erroneous telephone numbers (12.5%, n = 120) or nonresponse to repeated telephone and mail contacts (19.4%, n = 186). Approximately 2.0% (n = 18) refused to complete an interview at three months, and five participants had died.

Of those who were interviewed at three months, 39.9% (n = 238) were lost to follow-up at twelve months. Also at twelve months, more patients were unreachable because of incorrect or no telephone numbers (18.3%, n = 83), and many (13.0%, n = 59) did not respond to repeated phone calls. Nearly 2% (n = 9) refused to complete the twelve month evaluation, and twenty-one of the participants died during that time.

A total of twenty-eight patients in the intervention group and twenty-six patients in the control group reported at three months that they had quit smoking (Table 8.1). Patients in the intervention group had slightly higher self-reported quit rates (n = 28) for those interviewed and for all of those eligible for interview (10.0% and 6.1%) than in the control group (n = 26); (8.2% and 5.2%). However, at twelve months postenrollment, the self-reported quit rates for patients in the control group (n = 41) were higher than in the intervention group (n = 31) for those patients interviewed (17.1% vs. 14.4%) and for all patients eligible for interview (n = 39; 10.6% vs. n = 31; 8.4%). None of these differences were statistically significant.

At both the three and twelve-month follow-ups, roughly half of the self-reported quitters in each group provided saliva samples. At three months posttreatment, biochemically validated smoking-cessation rates ranged from 2.0% to 3.2% in the intervention group and 1.8% to 2.8% in the control group. Biochemical smoking-cessation tests suggest that nine patients from each group quit smoking (Table 8.2). At one year, the comparable rates were from 2.2% to 3.7% in the intervention group and 2.8% to 4.6% in the control group. Biochemical smoking-cessation tests suggest that eight patients from the intervention group and eleven patients from the control group quit smoking. These point estimates may represent entirely different respondents at distinct times. Deception rates in the intervention group ranged from 42.9% to 74.2% and from 31.3% to 73.2% in the control group, depending on the method of estimation used and whether those who did not provide saliva samples are eliminated or considered to be deceivers.

Three specific hypotheses concerning variables related to cessation were tested. First, it had been anticipated that individuals who smoked less than one pack a day would be more likely to quit following cessation counseling than would heavier smokers. The results supported this hypothesis. Lighter smokers, those who reportedly smoked less than twenty cigarettes per day, reported quitting at three and twelve months postenrollment with greater frequency than heavy smokers at the .05 level of significance, regardless of whether validated or unvalidated rates were used.

Second, it had been expected that patients who set target dates for cessation would be more likely to quit than those who did not. However, at both follow-up points there was no difference in quit rates between those who set target dates and those who did not. Third, it had been believed that more frequent clinic visits would positively impact smoking cessation. The number of clinic visits was examined to determine the cumulative effect of physician counseling. In general, individuals who visited a physician three or more times during their enrollment in the study had higher validated quit rates than those who visited a physician only once or twice. While the smoking-cessation rate increased with the number of clinic visits, this trend was not statistically significant, probably because of the small sample sizes.

Moreover, it had been anticipated that patients in the intervention group who continued to smoke during the study would report lower levels of cigarette consumption than patients in the control group, report more quit attempts, and be more likely to change smoking behavior. Patients in the intervention group smoked fewer cigarettes at three and twelve months than those in the control group; however, the differences were not statistically significant. Patients in the intervention group who continued to smoke at three and twelve months postenrollment reported more attempts to quit smoking than patients in the control group; again, however, the differences were not statistically significant.

The relationship of physician and patient gender was also examined. At three months postenrollment, male physicians were slightly more successful in counseling male patients to quit smoking than they were with female patients (1.3% vs. 0.0%). Female physicians were more successful counseling female patients to quit smoking than they were with male patients at three months (7.3% vs. 0.0%). However, at twelve months post-enrollment, male physicians were more successful in counseling their female patients to quit smoking than male patients (2.4% vs. 0.0%). Female physicians were much more successful with female patients than with male patients at twelve months (6.1% vs. 1.2%). Overall, female physicians were more effective counseling patients to quit smoking than were their male counterparts, particularly at three months (p < .05). The differential is due primarily to the effectiveness of female physicians with female patients. Female physicians seem to be more effective than male doctors teaching female patients about smoking cessation. The effects of gender on validated quit rates were mixed. Overall, female physicians were more effective than their male counterparts. Both sexes, though, were remarkably ineffective in getting male patients to quit smoking.

DISCUSSION

Several important methodological issues should be considered in relation to the results of this study. First, we experienced higher than expected loss-to-follow-up rates of 38% and 40%, respectively, at three and twelve months postenrollment. Possibly, the use of incentives would have improved the follow-up rates, given that many patients failed to return telephone messages. Second, we also experienced higher than expected weighted-average deception percentages (nonbiochemically validated and those who failed to provide saliva samples) of 55% at three months and 60% at twelve months. Finally, in spite of the intense recruitment efforts and the findings from the pilot study concerning rate of recruitment, in twenty-six months the desired sample size was not achieved. Significantly, 70% of the potential participants who were approached agreed to participate, but many did not return to the clinic for the study. Enrollment was most successful when recruitment occurred immediately prior to a clinical encounter that was part of the study.

It was estimated that a sample of 351 more patients at three months and 492 more patients at twelve months would be required to reach 80% power in the analyses. In fact, the actual power of the comparisons at three months was 61% and at twelve months only 26%. Consequently, insufficient power is a possible explanation for the failure to detect significant differences between the intervention and control groups.

In spite of the apparent lack of effect of the intervention, the following findings are noteworthy for future studies in similar populations.

1. All physicians in training in the targeted departments who were asked to participate in the study did so.
2. Eighty-seven percent of all eligible patients voluntarily enrolled in the study. Research assistants were on-site to identify and recruit study participants and encourage physician counseling. Other smoking-cessation studies would benefit if when recruitment occurred, counseling also commenced.
3. Seventy-three percent of the patients who were supposed to be counseled reported on exit interviews that they had actually been counseled by their doctors.
4. High loss-to-follow-up rates of 38% and 40% at three and twelve months, respectively, should be expected. Some attempt should be made to ensure that follow-ups are completed. One possible approach might be to use incentives following provision of required information.
5. Weighted-average deception rates (nonbiochemically validated and no saliva sample given) of 55% to 60% might be found at three and twelve months. It is, therefore, important to incorporate such validation as a routine part of any evaluation.
6. Future studies might evaluate the impact of provider ethnicity or gender upon the effectiveness of smoking-cessation messages.
7. Future projects should also attempt to identify a model for a successful intervener. What are his/her attributes?

Our experience also leads us to believe that a brief physician-delivered smoking-cessation message alone is not an effective method in a large, urban, public general hospital among adult African-American outpatients. We have demonstrated, however, along with others (Cummings et al. 1989a, 1989b; Glynn et al. 1990; Ockene et al. 1991; Kottke et al. 1992; McIlvain et al. 1992, 1995) training physicians in specific intervention approaches does increase the amount of communication with patients about smoking and smoking cessation. There is still room for improvement, as not all patients reported that they had been counseled. It is not possible to determine whether this was due to the physicians' lack of effort in this area or the patients' lack of attention to the information provided.

It is hardly surprising that one brief counseling session with a physician does not result in a permanent behavior change, but repeated advice, along with information in the media, legislated restrictions on smoking, and increased taxation, may combine to increase the likelihood that individual smokers will quit. The addition of other procedures, such as individual counseling by health educators, nicotine polacrilix, or nicotine transdermal patches, may lead to increased effectiveness of the physician's message. The use of focus groups to provide suggestions for future interventions should be an integral part of any evaluation.

ACKNOWLEDGMENTS

This research was funded by the National Cancer Institute, Contract #NO1-CN-65006.

NOTES

1.   The study group consisted of Alvin Thomas (principal investigator 1986–1989), Albert Niden (principal investigator 1989–1990), Bruce Allen, Jr. (project director 1986–1990; principal investigator 1990–1992), Virginia Li, Alfred Marcus, and Don Mareski of UCLA, research assistants, a data manager, and a secretary.

LITERATURE CITED

American Cancer Society. 1983. *A study of smoking behavior among black Americans.* New York: Evaxx.

Berman, B. A., A. K. Yancey, R. Bastani, et al. 1997 African-American physicians and smoking cessation counseling. *Journal of the National Medical Association* 89:534-542.

Brink S. G., N. H. Gottlieb, K. R. McLeroy, et al. 1994. A community view of smoking cessation counseling in the practices of physicians and dentists. *Public Health Reports* 109:135–142.

Burns, B., and J. P. Pierce. 1992. *Tobacco use in California, 1990–1991.* Sacramento: California Department of Health Services.

Cummings, S. R., T. J. Coates, R. J. Richard, et al. 1989a. Training physicians in counseling about smoking cessation: A random trial of the "Quit for Life" program. *Annals of Internal Medicine* 110:640–647.

Cummings, S. R., R. J. Richard, C. L. Duncan, et al. 1989b. Training physicians about smoking cessation: A controlled trial in private practices. *Journal of General Internal Medicine* 4:482–489.

Gilpin, E. A., J. P. Pierce, M. Johnson, and D. Bal. 1993. Physician advice to quit smoking: Results from the 1990 California tobacco survey. *Journal of General Internal Medicine* 8:549–553.

Glynn, T. J., M. W. Manley, and T. F. Pechacek. 1990. Physician-initiated smoking cessation program: The National Cancer Institute Trials. In *Advances in cancer control: Screening and prevention research*, ed. Paul F. Engstrom, Barbara Reimer, and Lee E. Mortenson, 11–25. New York: Wiley-Liss.

Jarvis, M. J., H. Tunstall-Pedoe, C. Feverabend, et al. 1987. Comparison of test used to distinguish smokers from nonsmokers. *American Journal of Public Health* 77:1435–1438.

Kottke, T. E., R. N. Battista, G. H. DeFriese, et al. 1988. Attributes of successful smoking cessation interventions in medical practice: A meta-analysis of 39 controlled trials. *Journal of the American Medical Association* 259:2882–2889.

Kottke, T. E., L. I. Solberg, M. L. Brekke, et al. 1992. A controlled trial to integrate smoking cessation advice into primary care practice: Doctors helping smokers, round III. *Journal of Family Practice* 34:701–708.

Li,V. C., T. J. Coates, L. A. Spielberg, et al. 1984. Smoking cessation with young women in public family planning clinics: The impact of physician messages and waiting room media. *Preventive Medicine* 13:477–489.

Manley, M. W., R. P. Epps, T.J. Glynn. 1992. The clinician's role in promoting smoking cessation among clinical patients. *Medical Clinics of North America* 76:477–494.

McIlvain, H. E., J. L. Sussman, M. A. Mannus, et al. 1992. Improving smoking cessation counseling by family practice residents. *Journal of Family Practice* 34:745–749.

McIlvain H. E., J. L. Sussman, C. Davis, and C. Giblet. 1995. Physician counseling for smoking cessation: Is the glass half empty? *Journal of Family Practice.* 40:148-152.

Miller, B. A., L. N. Kolonel, L. Bernstein, J. L. Young, Jr., et al., eds. 1996. *Racial/ethnic patterns of cancer in the United States 1988–1992.* NIH Publication No. 96-4104. Bethesda, MD: National Cancer Institute.

National Cancer Institute (NCI). 1998. Fact Sheet on Smoking and Cancer. Communication by e-mail from Margaret Reh to Diane Weiner, May 22.

Ockene, J. K., A. Adam, L. Pbert, et al. 1994. The physician-delivered smoking intervention project: Factors that determine how much the physician intervenes. *Journal of General Internal Medicine* 9:379–384.

Ockene, J. K, J. Kristeller, R. Goldberg, et al. 1991. Increasing the efficacy of physician-delivered smoking interventions: A randomized clinical trial. *Journal of General Internal Medicine* 6:1–8.

Ockene, J. K., J. Kristeller, L. Pbert, et al. 1990. The physician-delivered smoking intervention project: Can short-term interventions produce long-term effects for a general outpatient population? *Health Psychology* 13:278–281.

Ohlin, P., B. Lundh, and H. Westting. 1976. Carbon monoxide blood levels and reported cessation of smoking. *Psychopharmacology* 49:263–265.

Russell, M., C. Wilson, C. Taylor, et al. 1979. Effect of general practitioners advice against smoking. *British Medical Journal* 2:231–235.

U.S. Department of Health and Human Services. (USDHHS). 1994. Surveillance for selected tobacco-use behaviors, United States, 1990–1994. *MMWR* 43:3.

Wingo, P. A., L. Ries, H. M. Rosenberg, D. S. Miller, and B. K. Edwards. 1998. Cancer incidence and mortality, 1973–1995: A report card for the U.S. *Cancer* 82(6):1197–1207.

Table 8.1
Self-Reported Quit Rates by Study Group for Patients Interviewed and for All
Patients Eligible for Interview

Study Group	Intervention	Control
Time Period	**Three Months**	**Three Months**
Number Interviewed	279	318
Number Who Said They Quit	28	26
Quit Rate	10.0%	8.2%
Number Eligible	457	503
Number Who Said They Quit	28	26
Quit Rate	6.1%	5.2%
Time Period	**One Year**	**One Year**
Number Interviewed	216	240
Number Who Said They Quit	31	41
Quit Rate	14.4%	17.1%
Number Eligible	369	387
Number Who Said They Quit	31	39
Quit Rate	8.4%	10.6%

Table 8.2
Biochemically Validated Smoking-Cessation Rates for Patients Interviewed and for
All Patients Eligible for Interview

Study Group	Intervention	Control
Time Period	**Three Months**	**Three Months**
Number Interviewed	279	318
Number of Validated Quitters	9	9
Quit Rate	3.2%	2.8%
Number Eligible	457	502
Number of Validated Quitters	9	9
Quit Rate	2.0%	1.8%
Time Period	**One Year**	**One Year**
Number Interviewed	216	240
Number of Validated Quitters	8	11
Quit Rate	3.7%	4.6%
Number Eligible	369	387
Number of Validated Quitters	8	11
Quit Rate	2.2%	2.8%

Chapter 9

It Works! Breast Cancer Programs for African-American Women

Bettye Green and Ellen Werner

U.S. breast cancer incidence and mortality rates prior to the 1980s reinforced the belief that breast cancer is a white woman's disease. Over the life span, white women continue to have a higher incidence of breast cancer, but the incidence under age forty-five is higher in blacks (Ries et al. 1994). Since 1980, the age-adjusted annual mortality rates at all ages and age-specific death rates under age sixty-five have been higher among blacks than whites (Ries et al. 1994). African-American women have higher rates of late-stage disease at diagnosis and lower five-year survival rates (Wells and Horm 1992).

A major challenge to the public health system has been to raise awareness of breast cancer risk among African-American women and to remove barriers to health care utilization.

The health care system has an equally challenging task: to provide diagnostic, treatment, rehabilitation, and support services to minority women who traditionally have been underserved by that system. Breast cancer advocates, health care providers, and university-based researchers have attempted to meet these public health and health care challenges by organizing groups of breast cancer patients and survivors and by developing and implementing breast care programs targeting African-American women. The purpose of this chapter is to describe unique programs that have been developed to address the needs of African-American women with (or at risk for) breast cancer, to identify characteristics of successful projects, and to provide guidelines for organizers.

Information about the programs comes from semistructured and in-depth interviews the authors conducted with program organizers and providers of breast care services. Most interviews were conducted in person, although several were conducted by telephone. All respondents were informed prior to interviews that neither they nor their programs would be identified by name or location.

CASE REPORT 1: DR. A's UNIVERSITY-BASED PROGRAM

Dr. A organized a hospital and university-based program in a large urban area. The program started in the hospital, with the goal of meeting breast care and education needs of the entire community. Its major purposes are to provide breast cancer screening, education, and training in breast care and the use of the health care system. The program staff act as liaisons with the health care system. The hospital continues to support, fund, and house this program.

Dr. A's forte is public presentations, during which she relates experiences of African-American women and survivors. She stresses the value of outreach efforts: "[You] need to know more than just your material"; you need to know the target audience. She is currently developing an interventional guide for self-help programs.

Dr. A has observed that when people initiate breast cancer programs, they neglect to use tools and programs that are already available. They do not build an infrastructure or become familiar with methods of established programs. Rarely do people use evaluation tools to monitor program progress and detect problems.

She says, these are "good-hearted people who don't know how to do it" (i.e., establish a program), and they are not necessarily lay people. The main problems are lack of experience in developing and implementing health programs, and lack of awareness of national programs, such as those of the American Cancer Society. These problems can be overcome by becoming familiar with existing programs and tailoring them to fit local needs.

Dr. A says that monetary support is her major concern and that "sustained support is the issue. There should not be gaps in funding." Once a program begins, "it will disappear unless it's taken over by a major health program."

Dr. A sees no racial problems in her hospital-based program, yet, she says, African-American women are "not at the table" when breast cancer is discussed at the local, state, and national levels. The problem is that they are "not invited, not welcomed. [Other] people think they don't have skills; African-Americans feel that way, then they get turned off." "Talking down" is still a problem when other people work with African Americans; this is an age-old interaction in which whites talk to African Americans in a way that makes them feel stupid or as if they do not understand what is being said. Financial problems may also prevent many African-American women from "coming to the table"; they do not have the "financial flexibility to serve at the table, to take time off from work, or to [delegate] their family obligations."

In an ideal world, Dr. A would make sure that a breast cancer program was structured to include follow-up to diagnose and treat women, and mechanisms to cover costs of procedures for women who cannot pay. She would want the program to incorporate the continuum of care, education, and a paid staff. She recommends that a program be housed in a medical facility or clinic. Outlying or satellite sites should send patients to the clinic, and they should be part of an established health care plan.

CASE REPORT 2: MS. K'S HOSPITAL BASED-PROGRAM

Ms. K works in a hospital in a medium-size Midwestern city. She worked with hospital staff and breast cancer survivors to begin this program in 1993, because she recognized a disproportionately high breast cancer death rate among local African-American women. The program's purposes are to promote breast cancer awareness, communicate effectively with African-American women about the importance of screening and early detection, and to provide mammography. Although the program emphasizes screening, it provides all services for breast care, although not funding for those services. Ms. K continues to manage the program, with the help of a coordinator.

This program receives funding from various sources. The hospital provides financing, equipment, materials, and facilities. The community has a "tithing" program that donates funds. Ms. K and program staff secured several grants.

The program at Ms. K's hospital is designed to reach underserved African-American women, especially older women. Local physicians, religious organizations, and other hospitals refer women to the program and donate services for women who cannot pay for treatment.

The hospital-based program run by Ms. K provides a continuum of breast care to underserved women. If a woman's mammography screening is negative, she is recontacted in approximately twelve months for rescreening and counseling. If a mammogram is positive, the woman is called by the nurse coordinator, who arranges for any appropriate diagnostic procedures and treatment. The nurse coordinator organizes surgical treatment, and the woman is provided with help from the nurse and support group. Local physicians, other health care professionals, and nurses make their services available.

Ms. K felt pressure "to succeed . . . [and] did not want the head hospital administrator to say it did not work." She feels that when the program began African-American women were not represented locally when breast cancer issues were discussed, but that they are now. However, Asians and Hispanics are still excluded from the dialogue. African-American women can, Ms. K says, unite to express their concerns about cancer issues, but it "takes a lot of work." She thinks that scientists should recognize that they do not have African-American representation in clinical cancer studies. There is "no program designed for African-Americans; there needs to be more done."

Ms. K believes that initial distrust among the target population had to be overcome before women would participate fully in the program. She believes that "truthfulness, availability, and consistency" are important characteristics of program staff. Those qualities communicate the message that staff and the program are there to serve and will not let the African-American breast cancer patient slip through the cracks of the health care system.

Technology can be a barrier. Small organizations like Ms. K's cannot afford sophisticated equipment and computers. When they interact with larger or national organizations, they need hard copies of documents; their clients do not have access to home computers.

One struggle the program had to surmount was division of power within the hospital. It was housed in a department responsible for community outreach, which is separate from the hospital's cancer division office. "Once the program took off, both [departments] wanted credit" for it. With the administration's lack of unanimity about the program's organizational position, the "program was caught in the middle."

There was an initial misunderstanding about roles. The hospital's perspective was that a medical person should lead the program. However, women in the community thought the coordinator should be a lay health worker. Thus far, the two coordinators have been nurses who are African American, and this disagreement is no longer an issue. Ms. K believes that the nurse coordinator's position could have been more effective in the beginning had more money been available to fund her time, private office, and expenses.

Ms. K's program has been very successful in increasing the number of African-American women who are screened for breast cancer and receive appropriate follow-up care after positive mammograms. African-American women in the community "have gotten the message" that they are at risk. Ms. K has not felt that people or organizations wanted to regress to times when African-American women were ill served by the health care system, or that anyone involved wanted this program to fail. Ideally, Ms. K would have established the nurse coordinator's leadership at the beginning of the program.

CASE REPORT 3: MS. S'S UNIVERSITY-BASED PROGRAM

Ms. S initiated and organized a comprehensive breast cancer program that emphasizes screening yet provides education, training, and access to health care services. This mobile van program is based at a large, urban university that has a major medical school, hospital, and managed-care organization.

The purpose of the program is to provide comprehensive breast care services, including diagnosis, treatment, and support, "so [that] no woman falls through the cracks." Ms. S realizes that in this first year it will not be able to cover the costs of all the services it is providing, so the program will run a deficit. A foundation has promised to cover any shortfall at the end of the year. Ms. S believes that the only reason the mobile mammography program would go "belly-up is lack of support."

A marketing director was hired at the beginning of the program. She resigned after the first year and will not be replaced. There was not a good "fit" between her and the target communities; whether this was because she was white or because she had a business and marketing, rather than health, orientation cannot be determined. The "patient navigator,"[1] an African-American social worker, is well received by program participants. In this program, the patient navigator guides a client through the process of obtaining a mammogram.

A local television station airs public service announcements and special-interest stories about Ms. S's program. Staff members work with popular African-American radio stations and ask church pastors to announce the program's van schedule. Program staff have joined a community business partnership and attend its meetings. They work with advisory neighborhood committees, volunteer with food distribution, and train health liaisons. The program recently established an interinstitutional cooperative agreement with a neighboring university.

The biggest problem of the university-based mobile van program is insufficient numbers of women getting mammograms at scheduled sites. Ms. S and staff have struggled with this problem but do not have a solution. They will schedule a visit in a community, but "people in charge of the site don't get women, or don't get enough women" to come for mammograms. Ms. S lets the van go to a scheduled site even if only "six or seven" women have appointments, in the "hope that word of mouth helps later." "No-shows" compound the problem. Telephone calls to remind women do not help. Ms. S and staff wonder if they should schedule two women for each time slot, risking having women wait, or "overbook" by 10% to prevent down-time for the mammography unit and staff. They are looking for solutions, because the underbookings and no-shows waste resources.

Ms. S attributes a part of the problem to "getting people in the community to trust" the university-based program. The university did not have a good reputation for working in or with underserved communities prior to the van program. The communities' perspective was that the university was "coming in to tell them that [they] need a service that [the] community doesn't know it needs." Program staff did not conduct initial focus groups to determine the communities' needs or perceptions.

The program has nonetheless been successful in reaching underserved women. It has screened more women than they anticipated. In the first year of the program, 1,400 mammographic screenings were provided to underserved women in the city, a number greater than the yearly total in several states. Six women were diagnosed with breast cancer, all of them were asymptomatic.

These six signify a success: diagnosis at an asymptomatic stage is early-stage disease, and these women have a greater probability of long-term survival. The van program received an award from the local public health association, and "people from all over the country [are] calling to see how it runs." The staff works four days a week for ten hours a day. Ms. S is planning to hire another half-time technician.

Aside from underestimating "no-shows," Ms. S believes, she should have done more outreach with the target population instead of relying on what community leaders said during the planning stage. Hospitals in the underserved communities thought that the van did not belong there. Ms. S worked with pastors, who invited the van to visit their communities. The patient navigator goes to the same community meetings as staff from other hospitals and is "out in the neighborhood."

Women have to come to the university medical center for additional mammographic views. The program allows them to get vouchers for taxicab rides to the university medical center where they receive diagnostic and treatment services. The community hospitals "have to bribe their physicians to take on indigent patients, whereas [the university medical center] can handle" them.

Ms. S, who is white, realizes now that they "should have added African-American women leaders . . . up front." It has taken time for people to catch on to the program, which now has relationships with several racial and ethnic groups. Ms. S did not feel pressure because of race. She had established alliances with "a lot of community people [who] invited the van" and had been "given entree into the community." She has communicated with African-American women and groups by starting a local women's cancer coalition and working with institutions, ethnic groups, the Council for Aging Black Women, the YWCA, a local chapter of the American Cancer Society, neighboring universities, and a local foundation. The patient navigator is developing a directory of community resources. Ms. S's theme in working with people is "share[,] . . . do not duplicate." All six breast cancer patients diagnosed through the van program joined a support group, although "African-American women [have been] reluctant to come to support groups." The breast care center at her university has one group for African-American and one group for Latina women.

Ms. S says, "Yes, African-American women can unite on cancer issues, as evidenced in the local women's cancer coalition." However, they "are not worried about cancer." They worry about "daily survival, and put themselves last" (see Kagawa-Singer and Maxwell, Jones et al., in this volume). Mammography-promotion messages must take into account that this target population "will use services if it is not a bother." They have "other priorities; if [something] isn't broken, don't fix it." Therefore, the program is trying to send the message to low-income, underserved African-American women that their health is an important issue. "By making [mammography] accessible, it is harder for them not to do it."

Ms. S's program refers African-American women to NCI clinical trials, and she says that researchers are "absolutely" trying to recruit minority women. She and her staff research NCI protocols to determine if their patients are eligible. Staff have to "reassure [patients] that this [is] not another Tuskeegee."[2]

If Ms. S. had to start again with what she knows now, she would have hired an African-American woman for community outreach. She did not realize that race was as big an issue as it is. It took eight months to hire the patient navigator, who should have been in place at the start of the program to help establish working relationships with community members. After three years, the program will need other sources of funding in order to continue.

CASE REPORT 4: MS. L'S SUPPORT AND EDUCATION PROGRAM

Ms. L is a breast cancer survivor who organized her program three years ago to unify African-American women with breast cancer. This program links African-American breast cancer patients and survivors throughout several regions of the country. The "main reason for the program is survivorship." It offers support and educational services.

Its "commitment comes from [their] spirit." Its major hurdle is grant-writing skills and access to grant money; Ms. L attributes the program's lack of growth to a lack of funding. Currently, it is exploring ways of applying for and obtaining grants, and it would welcome help with the application process. It has "no funding but [is] going along anyway." Volunteerism and contributions of personal time and resources are the backbones of this program, which targets African-American breast cancer survivors

Ms. L's program operates on a shoestring. It is able to print and distribute brochures and pamphlets. Ms. L. is credited by people who know her as handling and dispensing money very efficiently. She is cautious about long-distance telephone calls and faxes, and she asks people, if they have the funds, to call her instead.

The group does not provide linkages with the health care system. Ms. L and her members do, however, assist breast cancer patients who feel that they are being ignored by their physicians, are not being treated appropriately, either medically or interpersonally, or have a problem that is not being handled adequately by their physicians. In those cases, Ms. L or another survivor will call the physician and intervene. They empathize with patients who are exasperated but too tired to pursue answers or be their own advocates.

Ms. L has met resistance "getting blacks to the table to discuss cancer issues." She felt that a national educational project "would be good," but "[she] got no help. Breast cancer puts everyone in the same boat; it is an equalizer." She felt "disappointment when [she] saw that there were still racial lines" in the way the health care system treated her. She felt that cancer should have eliminated all racial lines.

CASE REPORT 5: MS. M'S PROGRAM TO ADDRESS UNMET NEEDS

Ms. M is a breast cancer survivor whose program offers breast care training, education, advocacy, and referrals. Ms. M started this program in 1989, because she felt that policy decisions did not have input from African-American women. Another woman now directs the program, since Ms. M's involvement with other breast cancer organizations and national groups has grown. This program has been successful in obtaining grants and financing through consultation work and fund-raisers.

Ms. M's program targets low-income African-American women and benefits from financial and programmatic support from other community organizations and leaders, men's groups, religious organizations, and health care providers.

The staff of Ms. M's program use local media, brochures, fliers, and presentations to community groups to promote breast cancer awareness and health. They have held press conferences and perform community outreach, especially at local churches. They recommend working with ministers, inviting them to breakfasts, arranging with them for one-to-two-minute presentations during services, sending flowers to sick community members, and setting up booths at churches. These activities acquaint church members with the program staff and educate them about breast care. Program staff are then in a position to gain cooperation from church members and invite them to participate in screening. Ms. M's program does not provide linkages to other services, although it helps women with referrals to physicians.

Ms. M describes several obstacles that her group had to overcome, although she says they were conceptually challenges—she "didn't know they were struggles. [She] naturally thought these were things that had to be worked through." Funding was an initial barrier, although she has now raised money through various activities. Ms. M and her staff have found that other women's groups are competitive, which initially hindered her group. The larger issue, though, was "getting women to participate. Why didn't they? They were totally disinterested. Why [were we] bothering them with this? That [attitude] had to be overcome."

Ms. M considers her major achievement to be "the way I have been able to involve other women in breast cancer." Her mistake at the beginning, she says, was that she lacked "a plan of action." She "never thought [her program] would be this big [and] thought it would have blown over." As part of her group's growing pains, it needed to learn how to manage resources.

She also recognized the need to organize people in such a way that they can use their skills and get extra training. She started a leadership support group and established educational programs to "teach lay people how to go out into the community." Her program has professionals working on projects and a formal program for African-American women. Her "greatest joy [is the] rallying of African-American women around the country." Ms. M feels that she and her breast cancer program have had a great deal of support.

Ms. M felt pressure to succeed and was overwhelmed by it. She "had to stop, take a step back, and reevaluate; [she was] taking on too much." She communicates regularly with other African-American women and groups about breast cancer but does not think they have adequate representation when breast cancer issues are discussed. Participation at the state and national levels costs money. Breast cancer survivors whose jobs are not in the health field may feel that other people "at the table" are more qualified to discuss breast cancer issues. Breast cancer advocates have voiced their concerns about feeling undertrained and undereducated at the beginning of their involvement in breast cancer advocacy, and about their need for more education in order to deal with scientific issues. National institutions, such as the NCI, want a spokeswoman who can represent a major organization and voice their constituents' concerns.

Ms. M does not feel that there has been an effective attempt to get African-American women into clinical cancer trials. "A lot of physicians do not make referrals [to clinical trials]. Education is of utmost importance [to help] the physician understand [he/she] must get women into trials [and] to educate women about opportunities to get into trials." Women in Ms. M's program need help getting treatment; they are not enrolling in NCI trials or protocols.

In an ideal world, Ms. M would make sure that the infrastructure was developed before starting a group and would identify funding sources in advance.

CASE REPORT 6: MS. T'S HOSPITAL-BASED PROGRAM

Ms. T is a breast cancer survivor. She is the president of a breast cancer support group that, in addition to providing support, promotes breast cancer advocacy, training, and education. A local African-American male physician, Dr. R., started the group in 1988 and continues to act as its director and mentor. The group's mission is to inform African-American women of the need for breast self-exam, clinical breast exam, and mammography and to promote breast cancer advocacy among and for African-American women. They have not yet received funding, except from the physician-director and Hadassah, a Jewish women's organization. The physician-director provides dinner at evening meetings, which women attend directly from work.

The members of Ms. T's program are all African-American women, of various ages. Quite a few husbands attend their meetings; they "come faithfully with their wives." In response to the authors' question, "How did you get them involved?" Ms. T answered, "They started coming to support their wives and they continue to come." There are five men who regularly attend meetings and health fairs. One of the husbands helps them with computers and Internet access.

Although this support group relies on word of mouth among women in the community, it has used two special publicity strategies. First, it has worked with the state Department of Transportation to get a group license plate. It will display their group's name and logo, and it will stimulate funding. Second, they did a "portrait of hope display," which included a group picture of survivors. The display was supported by the local American Cancer Society chapter and was sent to all local shopping malls.

Ms. T is very positive. It was the only African-American support group in the state, and women were not aware it. Aside from a lack of breast cancer awareness and knowledge, this group had to overcome informational barriers. It started as a "small group [and is] beginning to grow because of outreach. People come to [its] seminars, conferences and fairs. [Its] name is getting out." Lack of funds inhibits it from doing all it could do. One thing it tries to do is "keep women involved. [Early in the program,] each meeting, twenty to thirty women came and the next meeting, another twenty to thirty different women came. Now, they are coming together, and the same women are coming. [In the beginning] a lot were dying; they were diagnosed so late, a lot of young women."

Dr. R, the originator, attends support group meetings. He has brought in plastic surgeons, helped to plan meetings, and educated women at the meetings. According to Ms. T, "Anything he thinks women need to be aware of, he'll inform them. If he can't come, he sends his wife. He provides meals because some women come straight from work. He is an unsung hero."

Ms. T's group has submitted grant applications, but it has not been awarded any monies. She does "not know if [she] didn't have a project worth funding. They need help with grant writing. [It was] not necessarily because of race that [it was] turned down." She feels that they need more education to write a fundable grant. She says that the message about breast cancer risk and screening for African-American women is hindered by "the perception of breast cancer as a white woman's disease, a rich white woman's disease. It's a stigma for black women, a religious stigma." The religious belief is that if one sins, she will get an illness. African-American women are still not being adequately informed; there is still ignorance about breast cancer.

Ms. T stresses the need for more education. There is a need for more breast cancer education for African-Americans, formal education for young people, and more African American oncologists. Hospital staff that serve African Americans need to learn how to make this population feel comfortable in clinical trials, by first establishing trust, being scrupulously honest, and adhering to the highest research ethics. More African-American young people need to become educated as researchers.

CONCLUSIONS

The authors appreciate the honesty in program organizers in describing their programs and problems they encountered. In the context of developing, evaluating, and revising programs, this information is instructional and reflects lessons learned. Subsequent programs can benefit from their experiences. On the basis of information from the interviews and our personal and professional experience with health programs, we offer guidelines and caveats to potential program organizers.

Establish Infrastructure

Have all of organizational and administrative plans well thought out before starting your program. Many minority health programs are conceived by committed people with a desire to correct a problem. However, commitment and desire are not sufficient to make a program succeed. You need to determine what the program will do, and how. Preexisting programs can be used but should be tailored to meet the specific needs of your locality and your target population. If you cannot find enough African-American health care professionals to work on the program, recruit lay health workers. Consider using a "buddy system," teaming professional and lay health workers. The professional can be a "background" person, who will help the lay health workers keep the program's content and methods consistent with best practices in breast care programs.

Do not depend on established community leaders to help the program gain acceptance. Often African-American leaders do not have as large a following as you might assume, nor can they speak for other people. Identify your own community liaisons. Visit a community center, see who runs it, and talk to that person. Go to a site or facility that you might want to involve in the program. Find the person who seems to have a following and ask them to join you. Do not hesitate to become part of a group with whom you want to work; you need their acceptance.

By networking in the community, you can find out where you will get your strongest support. Who takes people to doctors' offices? Who helps deliver meals on wheels? The person who will help with your program is someone who is already doing work in the community.

Find Sources of Funding

Learn about government and foundation grants. Talk freely about funds with anyone who is interested in your program. Communicate the idea that this program cannot run on commitment and desire alone. People often take the existence of programs for granted, and they do not experience the frustrations of lack of money. Keep talking money, and people will get the idea that you need help finding funds. When you have seed money, use some of it to develop a plan to secure sustaining funds. Develop a plan for short and long-term funding to cover costs of personnel, facilities, supplies, equipment, telephone, delivery services, fund-raising activities, and other administrative overhead.

If you plan to apply for grants, locate a grant writer. If you plan to request funds from a foundation or organization, become acquainted with someone from the organization and work with him or her. If you plan to collaborate with experienced researchers or health care providers in universities or health facilities, be very clear about the program's financial needs and work up a detailed budget.

Ask yourself: What do you have to give in exchange for the money? Find out about your obligations to donors and funding organizations. You are accountable to them and to all stakeholders in the program. You may receive donations with no contingencies, though usually there are requirements. You may be obligated to write a report, give a presentation, or open the program's books to scrutiny. Consider naming donors as cosponsors. Learn how to keep records, if you do not know already. Capacity-building programs are held throughout the country. Enroll, implement procedures, and follow through on all your obligations.

Have a budget and an accounting system. Assume that the program will be audited and that you will have to show how the money has been spent. Keep receipts; you have to know where your money is going. This is part of how organizers and donors will evaluate the program. Did you use your money wisely? Donors are more willing to give money if they see that it is being, and has been, spent wisely. Be sure to match program goals and spending.

Stress Education

Find out about other breast cancer programs and determine if they have any components that you can borrow. Become educated about the basics of breast cancer: the epidemiology of the disease, the clinical characteristics and subtypes, diagnostic procedures, and treatment options.

Learn enough to be comfortable talking about the disease with professionals and lay people. If your program will employ lay people either as paid staff or volunteers, they must also be educated about breast cancer. A lack of knowledge can seriously undermine the program's credibility.

If you try to "put something over" on African Americans, you will lose all credibility with them, and you will not be able to recapture it. Be scrupulously honest. They will decide if they can trust you and if you know what you are talking about. Keep your credibility and reputation intact through education. Be prepared to educate others about your program. Be able to defend what your program is doing and to answer questions intelligently.

Allow Time

The program will need time to grow, mature, and gain acceptance, and you and program staff will need time to establish trust. Programs for African-American women must take into account a culturally appropriate time frame, which may differ from your time frame. Program staff should put energy and time into establishing trust on the part of community liaisons and the target population. There is a misconception among program organizers, including African Americans, that the target population automatically trusts. Good-hearted people often think that they will be trusted simply because they are African American.

Trust can be the biggest hurdle, and it may have nothing to do with you, your program, or the staff. There is a history that has to be overcome. African Americans retain memories of all other programs that failed or abruptly ceased operating (see also Jones et al. and Burhansstipanov, this volume). Previous programs have been wrenched from the community, and people assume that yours will be too. People may be thinking, "Why should I participate in this program? It'll be gone next week or next month."

Many programs are set up with such limited amounts of money that they cease operations without warning. When you seek funds, assume that the first year will be devoted to capacity building. Apply for capacity-building grants, to give yourself enough time to plan, begin implementing, and revising the program. In that first year, seek sustaining or comprehensive grants to continue the program.

Organizers can give a community the impression that their program will be permanent rather than temporary. If your program is limited in time for any reason, make that clear at the start and set your plans and goals accordingly. Be certain that program staff members are aware of the time frame. In the past, communities and target populations have felt that they were lied to because they did not expect programs to end when they did.

Administratively, it will take a year to establish your program. Emotionally, it will take six months for the program and you to establish trust and become accepted and liked.

Find the Right Location

Your program, services, and activities need to be housed and offered in the right places.

Consider your target audience, their ages, and the times of day when services and activities will be offered. Does the location have an open, relaxed, and friendly atmosphere? Does it feel like a comfortable and homey place? It can be offensive to some women to meet in a church.

Remember, the participants are not coming to you; you have to bring the program to them. Try to build mobility into the program. Try to minimize the number of activities that will be held in a hospital; that is a place for sick people, and the women may not feel comfortable there. Health care providers and researchers may be comfortable in a hospital, but minority women feel that they are being watched. Find a place where the women can wear casual clothes. African-American women believe they need to wear their good clothes to a health care facility in order to get good care. If they feel that way coming to program activities, they likely will stop coming when they have worn to them all their good clothes.

Schedule Convenient Hours

Consider the women you want to reach. They may have to get a babysitter. They may have to travel by bus or public transportation. They will not want to come at 8:00 A.M or 8:00 P.M. They are accustomed to being made to sit and wait in clinics as if their time was not important; they do not want to wait unless it is a matter of life or death. The best hours for starting an activity or service are 2:00 P.M. to 6:00 P.M. They will want to return home before dark, especially if they are elderly. Working women need activities after 4:30 P.M or even after 6:30 P.M.

Attitudes Can Facilitate Your Program Goals

Racial differences were not emphasized by respondents in our interviews. Non–African Americans and African Americans can work together, but the former must understand that they need African-American women to help them understand the issues and how to apply health practices in their communities. Scientists and researchers, regardless of their race, need to understand that African-American women are the experts: they know their communities, what will work, and what will not. They will team with people to improve health. Be sensitive that it may be a new experience for the African-American woman to put herself and her health first.

Like Ms. M, conceptualize your obstacles as challenges. If you make a mistake, take responsibility for it, and if appropriate, apologize. Be positive and have hope.

Finally, keep in mind these ten summary points.

1. Decide what your program purposes and goals are.
2. Identify the target population.
3. Identify your resources and get sufficient money to start the program, hire staff if you can, and recruit volunteers.
4. Develop a plan for sustained funding.
5. Develop a realistic timeline for planning, initial start-up, and full implementation. Include all activities, especially initial and sustained funding, accounting, and program monitoring.
6. Identify channels of communication for the target population, and plan publicity

and outreach activities and materials.
7. Identify and modify program materials from other sources.
8. Hold training sessions for staff and volunteers.
9. Allow enough lead time to develop, test out and revise the goals, budget, resource allocation, roles of staff and volunteers, acceptability of the program to the target population, and communication strategies.
10. Periodically evaluate your program and document its progress and problems for yourself, staff, and stakeholders.

ACKNOWLEDGMENTS

This project was supported by a grant from Bristol-Myers Squibb and United States Surgical Corporation. We are very grateful to these companies and to their staff members for arranging funding. We offer our heartfelt thanks to the women who participated in our interviews and provided the information that made this chapter possible.

NOTES

1. For more information on the patient navigator program refer to H. P. Freeman, B. J. Muth, and J. F. Kerner. 1995. Expanding access to cancer screening and clinical follow-up among the medically underserved. *Cancer Practice* (January–February) 3(1):19–30.
2. It is beyond the scope of this paper to explain the Tuskeegee experiment and its continuing legacy. Any reader who is unfamiliar with this atrocity can learn more about it from reading Vanessa Northington Gamble, "A Legacy of Distrust: African-Americans and Medical Research," *American Journal of Preventive Medicine* 9:35–38 and James H. Jones, *Bad Blood* (New York: Free Press, 1993).

LITERATURE CITED

Ries, L. A. G., B. A. Miller, B. F. Hankey, C. L. Kosary, A. Harras, and B. K. Edwards, eds. 1994. *SEER cancer statistics review, 1973–1991: Tables and graphs.* NIH Publication No. 94-2789. Bethesda, MD: National Cancer Institute.
Wells, Barbara L., and John W. Horm. 1992. Stage at diagnosis in breast cancer: Race and socioeconomic factors. *American Journal of Public Health* 82:1383–1385.

Chapter 10

Implementing Effective Recruitment Strategies for a Cancer-Prevention Trial in Older Hispanic Women: A Clinical Trial Model

Lovell A. Jones, Richard A. Hajek, Janice Allen Chilton, Angelina Esparza, Sarah Ann G. Garza, Rosie Gonzalez, and Maria Rocio-Moguel

This chapter outlines the experiences in the recruitment and retention of Hispanic participants into a clinical trial. The nutritional intervention study, *Compañeras Sanas* (Healthy Friends), was conducted as part of the Breast Cancer Nutrition Group at the University of Texas M. D. Anderson Cancer Center in Houston. In the recruitment of a cohort of postmenopausal Hispanic females, an approach was developed to meet more closely the needs of this understudied population so as to increase the success of the program. In this chapter we describe the most important aspects of this clinical trial intervention.

Cultural competency is specific to this study and the keystone of recruitment and retention rates. Cultural competency not only recognizes differences in culture but works to overcome any challenges that arise from these differences, by incorporating local knowledge and culture (see Burhansstipanov, in this volume).

BACKGROUND

This intervention trial was an outgrowth of a 1992 pilot study examining the role of of nutrition and breast cancer. It is widely accepted that a diet high in fat and low in fiber contributes to breast, colon, and liver cancer (Jones et al. 1995; World Cancer Research Fund 1997). However, the direct association of a low-fat diet with a reduction in breast cancer incidence is not well understood. One possible explanation may be the effects of fat and fiber intake on the blood hormones, such as estrogens. Estrogen is one of the most important intrinsic factors that influences breast cell growth, both normal and abnormal. Additionally, almost all common breast cancer risk factors can be associated with estrogen. Generally speaking, increasing your life-time exposure to estrogen would thus increase your breast cancer risks.

Based on current data, we know that women in Latin American countries have some of the lowest incidence rates for breast cancer in the world. Could dietary differences result in bioavailable estrogen changes, subsequently reflecting different risks and yielding distinct incidences of breast cancer? The objective of the study was to investigate this hypothesis. Being able to correlate changes in bioavailable estrogens through changes in dietary intake could help determine the direct role of dietary patterns in breast cancer incidence.

Our pilot study found very little difference in the plasma estradiol level between white, Hispanic, and African-American women, but we did observe a significant difference in the percentage of non-protein bound estradiol between postmenopausal African-American women (higher) and postmenopausal Hispanic women (lower) (Jones et al. 1995). There was also a difference in the percentage of estradiol bound to albumin in postmenopausal Hispanic women, which may be related to a decreased risk of developing breast cancer. Dietary fiber may also play a significant role in regulating bioavailable estrogen levels.

Hispanic women offer a unique and challenging opportunity to study the role of dietary fiber in regulating bioavailable estrogens. The typical diet of this population, especially among Mexican Americans, is high in fiber and high in fat (Borrud et al. 1989). Although we have established a link between a high fat diet and certain cancers, the breast cancer incidence rate for Hispanic women is less than that of white non-Hispanic women (Wingo et al. 1998). Dietary fiber from food intake is helpful in reducing cancer as well as in providing nutrients and both soluble and nonsoluble fiber not found in supplements. Even though Mexican Americans have a diet high in saturated fat, their dietary sources for protein tend to also to include foods that are high in dietary fiber (Borrud et al. 1989). This increased fiber may be a key to eliminating free estradiol from the body and to decreasing a potential risk for breast cancer. The challenge then is twofold: maintaining, perhaps slightly increasing, the dietary fiber from fruits and vegetables for this population, but also decreasing the amount of fat, to ensure a diet that is balanced and nutritionally sound. Our intervention investigated this precept.

A second issue that this intervention addressed is the method of planning, designing, and implementing a clinical trial with a minority group. Participation in clinical trials by minority populations has been limited at best. There are many reasons cited for low participation and even lower retention rates; however, we believe that fear, lack of understanding about research, and miscommunication rank highest. In order to combat these barriers, a new methodology was created that placed the central focus on the community. Through this community-focused model we were better able to accommodate cultural differences and to bridge the gap between the community and a large research institution.

Although this was a nutritional intervention, its behavior-modification aspect was extremely important. It was felt that in order to precipitate dietary changes a group setting would be most helpful. The idea of *compañeras* (close friends or companions) was an outgrowth of the idea of "comadres" (women who share godchildren, or are close relatives, or are very good friends), a system that has been a source of support for Hispanic women for generations. This social system laid fertile ground to assure the support need in a behavioral change model.

PHASE I: DESIGN AND ASSESSMENT

In the assessment of the original program (1992 study), some of the key issues had to be reevaluated. These included development of advisory groups, redefinition of the study population, assignment of clinical sites, and selection and training of personnel. Understanding and becoming knowledgeable about the Hispanic community was paramount in making appropriate modifications to the original design.

Community Service Network (CSN) and Study Advisory Board

A key element to community outreach was the development of a Community Service Network (CSN). The network served as advisors in evaluating the original design, and it offered concrete ideas on the most appropriate methods to reach our study population. Building a network of community contacts and resources can be a time-consuming process and one that is unique for each community. Advisory groups are important in developing a relationship, initiating entree into the community, and guiding researchers as to the best methods of recruitment.

In order to understand the need for such a group, it is important to understand the uniqueness of each community. A community can be defined by ethnic group, geographic location, common goals, or a combination of any of these factors. It is imperative that any advisor be familiar with the population, be knowledgeable about the resources available to the community, and play an active role in the community. The Community Service Network for *Compañeras Sanas* consisted of community advocates and leaders, primary health care providers located in that community, clergy, lay people, the city health department, and community health clinic directors, all from the Houston-area Hispanic community.

A secondary advisory group, the Study Advisory Board (SAB), is similar to the Community Service Network but more "hands-on". The Study Advisory Board comprised nurses, doctors, and administrators. Members were the professionals with whom the participants were already familiar and with whom they communicated on a regular basis. It may not be necessary to have both advisory groups; this can be determined by the size of the intervention and familiarity with a particular community.

A final note on this topic is that it is important that the membership of these advisory groups be based on the recommendations of the community. Advice from community liaisons, such as gatekeepers, can give ideas for influential representatives who might have a great impact on the community and be able to effect change.

Closer Definition of Study Population

As in other components of the intervention trial, it was important to reexamine our definition of our study population. This is particularly true when recruiting a diverse population, in this case Hispanics. In the planning phase of the *Compañeras Sanas* intervention, the targeted population was initially defined as postmenopausal Hispanic women with specific health criteria. However, once recruitment began it became quite evident that the eligibility criteria had to be adjusted.

Examining the diversity of the Hispanic population in Houston may be helpful for understanding why our focus changed. Houston has an extensive Hispanic community, so widely diverse that it would be difficult to describe in a blanket statement. This is probably the case in most large cities in which the population contains a myriad of cultures and subcultures. Socioeconomic and education levels, migratory patterns, and levels of assimilation are variables that must be considered when a cohort for a particular population is created. Although similarities may exist, subtle differences in customs and cultures could have a confounding effect on the outcome of a trial. We had to redefine our inclusion and exclusion criteria to reflect more closely the studied population in regards to literacy, economics, age, and geographic location. For example, unlike the pilot study, the *Compañeras Sanas* program had participants with fixed incomes. In examining an individual's motivation to change, we were concerned that basic primary needs not being met (shelter, food, clothing, etc.) might hinder dietary changes.

Selection of Clinical Site

It was the intention of the research study design to deliver this program in a community setting that would be easily accessible to the targeted community. Practical use of the Community Service Network and the Study Advisory Board helped us plan and accomplish this goal. On their advice, we recruited from areas of Houston that were heavily populated by Hispanics. These areas were primarily urban environments close to the central part of the city, where the average income level was reported to be lower or middle class.

The recruitment was done through mediating structures and community institutions (neighborhood clinics and senior programs). This method made routing participants much easier. Any participant who was qualified (on the basis of a phone interview) was instructed to attend the program orientation located closest to her; this way, a woman remained in her own neighborhood and community. This approach allowed us to gather enough candidates in one site to randomize. All these combined efforts led to the recruitment of over 300 candidates for initial screening and about forty randomized participants.

For a number of reasons, it was important to solidify all arrangements with participating agencies. The staff met with members of our advisory boards, who were instrumental in developing collaborative efforts with neighborhood centers. Using the advisors' contacts, we were able to establish a relationship with the clinic administration and staff. Such details were discussed as: Where will the nutritional classes be conducted? What will be the frequency of the meetings? By creating these mediating relationships in the beginning, recruitment was facilitated.

Transportation

Although the staff had previously considered some of the barriers, its meetings with administrators of multiservice centers, clinical directors, and CSN and SAB members elucidated additional issues. For example, advisors informed the staff that older Hispanic women do not like to travel at night: they are fearful of driving, or of being driven, at night in Houston, due to heavy traffic, inability to read road signs, and the like. Classes were thus held during the day. Additionally, potential participants frequently had limited transportation. Further consultations about the proposed study, with both advisory groups, made it clear that transportation to the Texas Medical Center for clinical exams would have to be addressed in order to ensure success. Funds were allocated to cover the cost of transportation between the Center and the clinical sites on clinical exam days. Additionally, to make the participants more comfortable, the same driver was assigned when possible; he could become familiar with the passengers, who would know him by name.

One issue that could not be overcome, due to budgetary constraints, was transportation to and from the nutritional classes. However, conducting these classes during the day and in local neighborhood centers helped alleviate this barrier for the majority of the participants.

Staffing

Successful recruitment is based on a trusting relationship between the research staff and study participants. Thus, the importance of this selection process should not be overlooked or taken lightly. The selection of personnel should be based not only on educational and professional experience but also on cultural sensitivity and competency. It is preferable, though not necessary, that staff members reflect the attributes of the study populations in race, ethnicity, gender, and cultural experience. By the same token, however, selecting an individual based solely on his/her ethnicity will not guarantee success. Belonging to a minority group will not automatically provide an individual with a special affinity for all minority populations. Unique skills might be required to meet the needs of a study population. For example, the ability to speak Spanish to monolingual participants was an absolute necessity.

Understanding the community members' thoughts and concerns was an imperative for us. The project team always exhibited an empathetic attitude. Traditional staffing may not offer sufficient manpower for the needs of minority and medically underserved populations. In developing the *Compañeras Sanas* program, the staff first had to understand the community ideas and views on nutrition and cancer. Staff also had to listen to the participants' questions and be respectful of their beliefs and concepts. Taking this additional time to evaluate, ask questions, and receive feedback was essential for developing a trust, credibility, and rapport with our participants. All of these qualities in personnel are important, and they can be achieved by an astute selection and proper training. As a result, problems and barriers that arose were viewed not as the participant's or group's shortcomings but rather as challenges that would require a more innovative approach.

Form Development and Translation of Materials

Proper delivery of educational information and collection of clinical trial data for this study was critical. All too often, investigators and staff members use medical terminology that does not effectively deliver the intended message to a lay audience. Materials should be developed with the audience in mind, ensuring that information is structured in the most appropriate form. This may mean that one not only considers literacy level and appropriate language but also takes into account any specific dialects and beliefs.

Translation and development of screening forms and educational materials occurred in the assessment and recruitment phases concurrently (Figure 10.1). In the assessment phase, we realized that most of the forms and educational materials had been created for a higher literacy level than that of the targeted population. Also, materials were not available in Spanish. Therefore, modification of forms and materials became an important part of the initial stages of the program.

To cite a more specific example, the research staff had to find or develop specialized dietary assessment tools that would accurately collect pertinent data. The two tools that were used were a food frequency questionnaire and a dietary food record. A food frequency questionnaire (FFQ) is a tool used by many studies to assess dietary intake. A food frequency questionnaire had been used in the 1992 pilot study. The questionnaire is a precoded form that supplies respondents with a list of sixty to 120 food lines, which may consist of a single food item (e.g., white bread) or of a group of foods having similar nutrient composition (e.g., English muffins, bagels, and rolls) (Teufel 1997). The original food frequency questionnaires had been formulated to test a standard middle-income "American" diet.

It was the consensus of the staff that modifications were needed. In recording proper nutrient intake, inaccuracies might arise among ethnic subgroups in the populations whose diet patterns differed markedly from those of the general population (Borrud et al. 1989; Coates and Monteilh 1997). In order to meet the objectives of this study, we incorporated the work of Dr. Cheryl Ritenbaugh, who had developed a modified version, the Southwest Food Frequency Questionnaire (SWFFQ) (Ritenbaugh 1995). The SWFFQ was developed for a Mexican-American population in the Southwest region of the United States. A nineteen-page questionnaire with 179 lines, it consists of both single-entry foods and food groups. It separates refried beans from baked or cooked beans and plain rice from Mexican rice. Dr. Ritenbaugh also advised that it would be best to administer the SWFFQ by oral interview, in view of the average low literacy level of her original study population; this proved to be an effective method for data collection for our population as well.

The major limitation of the food frequency questionnaire instrument is that it does not record details of an individual's diet (preparation, quantity, etc.). The food record is a more precise record of quantity, preparation, and consumption of specific food items. It is recorded over a shorter period of time, for three nonconsecutive days (a total of five times). This tool collects information that more closely reflects behavioral changes; accordingly, the staff had to ensure that the participants would completely understand it and be able to report reliable information.

On the basis of a standard food record collection form, a unique food record was created in both English and Spanish by our staff. Modifications were made to the record. Lines were enlarged to help the visually impaired. Visual aids (pictures) of traditional foods were also added. Additional space for noting the time of day that meals were eaten was included. Detailed and explicit instructions, with examples, were given to ensure that participants understood how to complete the forms properly and completely.

PHASE II: RECRUITMENT

It is well documented that recruiting study participants from minority communities in clinical trials is a daunting task. Research conducted by Swanson and Ward describes four general barriers to recruitment and participation: sociocultural, research, economic, and individual (Swanson and Ward 1985).

Sociocultural barriers include the long-standing fear and apprehension in minority populations of the clinical health care system, including its research aspects. This can be attributed in part to historical disenfranchisement from society in general and from health care systems more specifically. It would be erroneous for researchers to believe that such incidents as the Tuskeegee syphilis trial are merely history and have long been forgotten (see Moore, and Green and Werner, in this volume). They have in fact made a lasting mark in some communities. To combat this inherent distrust it is important to understand local history and address apprehensions with honesty and frankness. In this way, one can begin to approach these minority communities and be more likely to succeed in recruitment.

The second barrier is limited availability of research and data. Minority communities and the medically underserved are underrepresented in clinical trials and research. Medical investigations are often conducted in a restrictive manner, offering programs only at certain sites, certain hours, and to those who are insured. Related to this restriction is the temptation to generalize data from a nondiverse population to the general public. It is for this reason that results frequently do not fit all ethnic groups.

The third barrier is economics, including access to health care and health insurance. This problem has played a major role in the exclusion of certain populations. Many research protocols do not cover the additional expense of test and trial participation. If individuals do not have insurance or some other way of paying, their participation is not feasible. Additionally, as alluded to earlier in this chapter, if basic needs are not met there may be small motivation for participation in a program from which the participant gleans little direct benefit; research is no exception.

Finally, individual barriers, including personal thought processes about health and disease, should not be overlooked. Perceptions of disease and health vary from culture to culture. For example, many of the women who participated in our program believed that cancer is an external entity, that little if anything could be done if cancer was diagnosed, and that there was little chance for survival (see also Champion and Menon 1997).

However, it is important to note that it would be erroneous to label all minority groups as having a fatalistic attitude towards disease. Based on our experience, participants were eager to learn all preventative methods that would help decrease their risks. Incorporating the clinical concept of prevention can be a challenge when working with varied cultures. It is important to recognize, respect, and understand the belief system of any group rather than impose a standard, structured protocol that might not accommodate these views.

Orientation

This population was not familiar with clinical trials or research, so an effort was made to educate it. The first goal was to introduce the concept of research. Staff members appeared on televised broadcasts to explain the role of nutrition and its relationship to cancer risks. Simultaneously, a media campaign was started about the study. We took advantage of this opportunity to use citywide media in a program "kickoff" campaign. A number of local Hispanic celebrities and politicians participated. Using our Community Service Network, we were able to induce a number of contacts to lend their names and participation. We then concentrated our efforts primarily in minority-based media and Spanish-language stations. The use of electronic media for recruitment purposes was very effective. When the first televised feature aired, our office received a number of telephone calls from interested women (approximately 300!). As calls were received, our recruitment coordinator completed the preliminary screening over the phone.

Following the recruitment of these participants, an orientation to the overall study, as well as to the participants' role in the study, was given. The research staff explained the program in great detail in an open, frank, and educational environment. An orientation session is a great chance for the staff and participants to begin to develop a rapport through interpersonal, face-to-face communication. Potential participants were given the opportunity to see an informal presentation of the study (community presentation), and they were provided written information to share with family and friends. The primary face-to-face recruitment message addressed concerns that were determined to be salient: perceptions about embarrassment, the safety of radiation (in mammograms), pain, cost of participation, anxiety over screening results, lack of awareness about the importance of the screening exams, and views about diet in the prevention of cancer. The staff emphasized the importance of participation as a possible contribution to the health of future Hispanic generations, as well as one's own. By adopting healthier eating habits and sharing this information with their families, they could understand how research and prevention played a role in their own health and that of their loved ones.

A second component of our orientation was the completion of all necessary paperwork. This included distributing educational materials on which exams the participants might undergo, distributing informed consent forms, obtaining any pertinent demographic information (age, SES, etc.), and scheduling the first clinical exam if a participant was qualified. All materials were provided in applicable languages, in this case both English and Spanish, and in basic, simple terms. People with literacy problems may be found among all ethnicities, races, and classes; we were concerned that participants with low-income levels might also experience limited literacy and difficulty with processing some written information. To aid those with limited reading skills, all handouts were reviewed and visual aids were added as needed. Posters, diagrams, and pictures guided participants through the orientation. Participants were informed regarding expectations, benefits, and the amount of time each would have to commit.

Information omitted from these materials may later become a problem. For instance, participants were originally informed that the staff with whom they would have direct contact with would be female. This was case, with the exception of one physician, Dr. Pat Vehrs, the administrator of the TOBEC (total body electrical conductivity) exam. Later, one of the participants brought this issue to the attention of a Patient Coordinator. We quickly informed all other participants of this omission. Even though it may seem insignificant, allowing the participant to know all aspects of the study is important.

Correspondence

The staff kept in constant correspondence with the participants. This was done to ensure that participants were kept informed throughout the project and to remind them of class meetings, clinic exam dates, and other information. One problem was that participants commonly had interruptions in phone service (lines were disconnected). In addition to follow-up phone calls, therefore, letters of acceptance were sent to those who qualified. Reminder calls were also made the day before classes met and before clinical exams took place.

PHASE III: PARTICIPANT MANAGEMENT

Participant management is the final phase of our participatory intervention model. Interpersonal communication affects the success of recruitment, screening, and retention. In our study, the most direct patient contact took place during the phase from enrollment into the program to the clinical exams. For instance, staff individuals clarify correspondence and remind participants of their rights as volunteers while in the program. This focus on interpersonal communication increases adherence and compliance, as it establishes an "open door policy" between the participant and the research staff. If a participant is unclear on an idea or responsibility, she knows that she can call and speak directly to a familiar individual who can address the item and explain it in understandable terms.

Message Delivery and Reinforcement

The goals and objectives of the program are constantly reviewed with the participants. The staff felt that it was important that these women not only take an active role in changing their eating patterns but understand the possible benefits for themselves, their families, and future generations. Conversations a year later with many of the ladies who had completed the program showed that this message had been firmly planted. The idea of beneficial results for their families was a significant encouragement to participation; family is vital in the Hispanic community. We found that the women were also proud to contribute to the understanding of cancer and diet within their communities. The women understood that they could take steps in their lives that could have a direct effect on known risk factors for cancer and other diseases. This in turn would not only pique interest in participation but also, we hoped, increase adherence and decrease attrition. When later interviewed one participant proudly stated, "I have helped scientists discover ways to reduce the next generation's risk for developing breast cancer." A number of participants asserted that they would be willing to participate in future clinical trials. Thus, our goal was accomplished.

Patient Coordinators

Patient Coordinators are members of our staff who have direct and constant interactions with the participants. Their primary purpose is to assist participants, act as translators, offer support, and coordinate appointment scheduling. The Texas Medical Center, the largest medical center in the world, can be overwhelming to most visitors, which is often stated as a reason that people do not participate in clinical research. Therefore, as participants arrive to the Texas Medical Center for clinical exams it is imperative that our Patient Coordinators be at curbside to greet and accompany the women through their visit.

Patient Coordinators also act as patient advocates, ensuring that the volunteers are treated in a culturally sensitive and respectful manner. Once a rapport has already been established between the Coordinator and the participant, we felt, their needs were best met by communication with the same people. The function of the Patient Coordinator is an important component of a successful program. Patient Coordinators have become an important part of our retention strategy; the participants are very appreciative of the support and respect that they experience from them while in the study.

Participant Interaction

The women attended their clinical exams and nutritional sessions not individually but in groups. This practice was helpful not only in providing support but also in promoting cohesion within the group. The idea of *Compañeras Sanas* (healthy friends) was to promote an informal support group wherein participants would quickly form alliances and share ideas and concerns. The participants helped each other with information, thus becoming more independent from staff and taking an active role in prevention and health promotion.

CONCLUSION

The enrollment of minorities into clinical trials, especially prevention trials, has received special attention over the last decade. Attempts to enroll have met with failure most of the time. There are many reasons to account for the low accrual rates of minorities in clinical research. However, such attempts can be summarized in the following phrase: "If you always do what you always did, you will always get what you already got."

Compañeras Sanas exemplifies an idea set forth by Dr. Martin Luther King in 1963 regarding civil rights, an idea that rings true for the involvement of minorities into clinical trials: "If you want to move people, it has to be toward a vision that's positive for them, that taps important values, that gets them something that they desire, and it has to be presented in a compelling way that they feel inspired to follow."

Including communities in the research process makes recruitment and retention more successful. Our group has been mobilized in a direction that benefits their own community, their families, and ultimately future generations.

As Dr. Gilbert Friedell, Director of Cancer Prevention and Control at the University of Kentucky, once stated, "If the problems are in the community[,] . . . the solutions are in the community." This view was demonstrated by *Compañeras Sanas*.

Almost all people are concerned about their health and the health of their families. The issue is how best to approach each community to resolve health issues. Health in minority communities cannot be approached as a single issue; rather it should be addressed in a holistic manner. The holistic approach used by the staff took into account factors that influenced individuals' perceived need for health care.

What are the key elements in a successful recruitment and retention effort? Based on the experience of this study, they include the following: (1) creating a planning and supervisory committee that includes persons who represent the desired population; (2) including minority physicians or scientists in leadership roles in the study; (3) developing an early partnership with the community; (4) using a variety of appropriate health education and communication methods and capitalizing on the strengths of each; (5) employing culturally competent methods, procedures, and instruments to measure the trials success, and (6) realizing the need for sufficient funds and manpower to implement and complete the study. One word of caution with regard to the first two elements: neither the color of skin, nor genetic makeup, nor ability to speak a language guarantees that an individual will be sensitive to or even knowledgeable about a community that you have assigned them to represent.

From our experiences we hope that one can learn these crucial points: trust, respect, partnership, communication, and flexibility. Trust and respect is a two-way street. A true partnership has to be on an equal plane, and it can only be achieved via communication and the ability to be flexible with regards to the community.

ACKNOWLEDGMENTS

The Breast Cancer Nutrition Research group at UTMD Anderson Cancer Center would like to acknowledge and thank our sponsor, the Kellogg Company, for its support of this research. The generous contribution made by the Kellog Company has been the key in assuring that this program continues in and for the community.

LITERATURE CITED

Block, G., J. C. Norris, R. M. Mandel, and C. DiForgra. 1995. Sources of energy and six nutrients diet over low-income in Hispanic-American women and their children: Quantitative data from HHANES, 1982–84. *Journal of the American Dietetic Association* 95:195–208.

Borrud, L. G., P. C. Pillow, P. K. Allen, R. S. McPherson, and M. Z. Nichaman. 1989. Food group contributions to nutrient intake in white, blacks, and Mexican Americans in Texas. *Journal of the American Dietetic Association* 89:1061–1069.

Champion, V., and U. Menon. 1997. Predicting mammography and breast self-examination in African-American women. *Cancer Nursing* 20(5):315–322.

Coates, R. J., and C. T. Monteilh. 1997. Assessment of food frequency questionnaires in minority populations. *American Journal of Clinical Nutrition* 65S:1108S–1115S.

Delgado J. L., and National Hispanic Women's Health Initiative. 1997. ¡SALUD! A Latina's guide to total health: Body, mind, and spirit. New York: Harper Collins.

Jones, L. A., D. DiPaolo, W. Insul, C. David, D. Johnston, M. Follen-Mitchell, V. Vogel, A. Berkowitz, R. Shallenberger, and W. Klish. 1995. The effect of a low-fat diet on bioavailable estrogen levels in an ethnically diverse population. *Proceedings of the American Association for Cancer Research* 36:686.

Ritenbaugh, C. 1995. Personal communication.

Swanson, G. M., and A. J. Ward. 1985. Recruiting minorities into clinical trials: Toward a participant friendly system. *Journal of the National Cancer Institute* 87(23): 1747–1759.

Teufel, N. 1997. Development of culturally competent food frequency questionnaires. *American Journal of Clinical Nutrition* 65S:1173S–1178S.

Wingo, P., et al. 1998. Cancer incidence and mortality, 1973–1995. A report card for the U.S. *Cancer* 82(6): 1197–1207.

World Cancer Research Fund/American Institute for Cancer Research. 1997. Food, nutrition and the prevention of cancer: A global perspective. Washington, DC.

Figure 10.1
Venn Diagram Phases of Effective Recruitment Strategies for a Cancer Prevention Trial in Older Hispanic Women

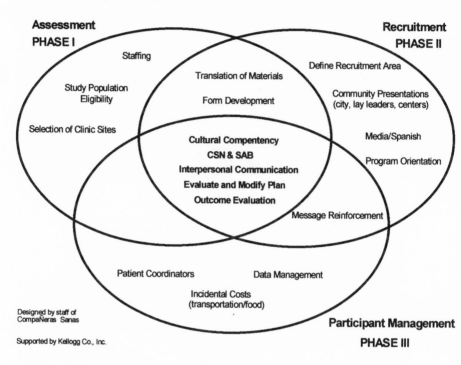

Assessment
PHASE I

Recruitment
PHASE II

Staffing

Translation of Materials

Study Population
Eligibility

Form Development

Selection of Clinic Sites

Define Recruitment Area

Community Presentations
(city, lay leaders, centers)

Media/Spanish

Cultural Compentency
CSN & SAB
Interpersonal Communication
Evaluate and Modify Plan
Outcome Evaluation

Program Orientation

Message Reinforcement

Patient Coordinators

Data Management

Incidental Costs
(transportation/food)

Designed by staff of
CompaÑeras Sanas

Supported by Kellogg Co., Inc.

Participant Management
PHASE III

Chapter 11

Native American Cancer Survivors: Agents for Change

Judith Kaur

This chapter will outline the history of cancer in Native Americans since the turn of the century, describe the patterns of cancer across the tribes today, and point to the important role of cancer survivors as agents for change. SEER data recently released shows that Native Americans have the poorest survival rate of any racial group in this country for cancer. Nonetheless, cancer survivors exist on every reservation, in every pueblo and urban enclave, and they are incredible resources for trying to change the survival rates for their people. This chapter will describe the empowerment of cancer survivors, barriers to detection and treatment and how to overcome them, the cultural aspects of cancer within native cultures, and the need for future interventions.

HISTORICAL PATTERNS OF CANCER IN NATIVE AMERICANS

There was a time, before the turn of the century, when it could truly be said that cancer was very uncommon among the indigenous populations of North America. Indeed, as recently as 1910 Levin stated that full-blooded American Indians *never* had cancer; medical journals found individual cases of cancer in American Indians to be reportable because of their rarity (Levin 1910). A 1930 article by Burton Lee in *Surgery, Gynecology and Obstetrics* reviewed the issue and asserted that there were rare verifiable cases of carcinoma in full-bloods but that the majority of cases occurred in mixed-blood Indians (Lee 1930). He postulated that the healthy lifestyle of traditional Indians might be responsible for the lower cancer incidence (he acknowledged, however, that many cases might be "undiscovered"). Among the "healthy habits" alluded to in this article were a longer period of nursing of infants, low incidence of gonorrhea, coarser natural foods, lower use of salt, less regular alcohol use, lighter eating habits, and increased physical exercise, compared to their European counterparts. The current guidelines published by the American Cancer Society for cancer prevention are: eat more fruits, vegetables, and grains; eat less high-fat foods and meats; be active and stay fit; drink less alcohol, if you do drink; and avoid tobacco product use (ACS 1996). It is intriguing to note how closely the traditional American Indian lifestyle parallels the recommendations from the American Cancer Society today for reducing cancer risk!

Creagan and Fraumeni reported on the basis of a series of 5,897 deaths from cancer in 1950–67 that there was still less cancer in both male and female Indians than in U.S. whites and nonwhites (1972). The *Journal of the National Cancer Institute*, however, in 1973 confirmed that some cancers were notably increased in incidence among U.S. Indians, including cervical cancer and gallbladder and biliary tract tumors, though cancers of the lung, breast, and bladder remained infrequent (Dunham et al. 1973). The high rate of gallbladder cancer in Southwestern tribes has been attributed to the known high frequency of gallstones and cholecystitis.

During 1960–69, 321 deaths attributed to cancer occurred among Alaska Natives (Eskimos, Indians, and Aleuts). The data was derived from the National Center for Health Statistics (Blot et al. 1975). The mortality of Alaska Natives from cancers of the nasopharynx, esophagus, kidneys, and salivary glands showed a significant increase over the Alaskan Caucasian population. Age-specific mortality rates for all cancers combined were generally higher among Alaska Natives than Alaskan Caucasians in both males and females. Most striking was the greater than tenfold excess of nasopharyngeal cancer.

A study based on a survey of epidemiological literature performed by Skye and Hampton in 1976 and published in the *Proceedings of the Third International Symposium on Detection and Prevention of Cancer* indicated that cancer was increasing in native populations and had a heterogeneous pattern. The most common cancers, such as that of the lung, breast, and colon, still, aparently had lower incidence rates among American Indians than in the general U.S. population. In contrast, cancers that were uncommon in the general population had higher rates in native people. These included cervical cancer, gallbladder cancer, hepatomas, and nasopharyngeal cancers.

The first bibliography of cancer in Native Americans and Alaska Natives from 1800 to 1989 was published by Justice in 1989 at the Native American Research and Training Center at the University of Arizona. Mahoney and Michalek updated the literature search for 1966–1994 with their publication in *Alaska Medicine* (1995).

THE INDIAN HEALTH SERVICE

The Indian Health Service (IHS) is the agency within the Department of Health and Human Services responsible for providing federal health services to American Indians and Alaska Natives. The Indian Health Service comprises twelve regional administrative units, called "Area Offices." IHS responsibilities extend to all or parts of thirty-five states known as "Reservation States." Reservation states are those with federally designated trust lands for tribes. This system integrates health services delivered directly through IHS facilities, purchased by IHS through contractual arrangements with providers in the private sector, and those delivered through tribally operated projects and urban Indian health programs.

According to the most current IHS statistical reports, cancer is now the second major cause of death in American Indians/Alaska Natives. In fact, in Alaska Native women cancer is now the *leading* cause of death (Lanier et al. 1996). These facts document a dramatic change since the 1950s, when cancer was ranked seventh among causes of death. There is wide variation in cancer incidence and mortality from region to region and tribe to tribe. It is therefore extremely difficult to generalize about cancer rates in American Indians/Alaska Natives. For example, while the overall mortality rate for breast cancer among AI/AN women is 42% *lower* than the all–United States rate, the Aberdeen, South Dakota, and Billings, Montana, area rates are actually *higher*. Studying the differences in cancer rates from tribe to tribe and region to region may offer important clues to the relative contributions of genetics, lifestyle, and environmental exposures.

DATA SOURCES

SEER

The Surveillance, Epidemiology, and End Results (SEER) data system was set up by the National Cancer Institute in 1971 to sample data on cancer incidence and mortality across the United States. A continuing project of the National Cancer Institute, the SEER program is responsible for monitoring the impact of cancer on the general population. SEER data from American Indian and Alaska Native populations involves only a small sample of the Southwestern tribes and Alaska tumor registry data. The first SEER data review showed an apparent lower incidence of cancer overall in American Indian and Alaska Natives but noted that the five-year mortality was significantly worse than that recorded for whites or blacks. Thus, while preliminary data suggested that American Indians were less likely to develop cancer in their lifetime, the corollary was that if they did develop it they were less likely to survive or to be cured at five years.

The latest SEER report confirms higher incidence rates for kidney, cervical, and for colorectal cancer (especially Alaska Natives) than for the all-races U.S. data (SEER 1996). The absence of a national cancer registry makes accurate data on cancer impact for AI/ANs hard to obtain. There are proposals to increase the representation of American Indians/Alaska Natives in the SEER registry for future data collection efforts.

State Health Department Statistics

The Indian Health Service is piloting projects that will cross-link tribal enrollment with state health department data and death certificates to capture accurate incidence and mortality data. Initial projects in California and Minnesota have shown significant variances, with major increases in both incidence and mortality due to cancer. Prior to the pilot project in Minnesota, cancer incidence data adequately representing populations of American Indians living in Minnesota were unavailable. Obtaining the incidence rates involved combining information from IHS, the Minnesota Cancer Surveillance System (a statewide tumor registry administered through the Minnesota Department of Health), and the Minnesota census of population and housing. Key findings included recognition that prostate cancer is now the most common invasive cancer affecting American Indian men in Minnesota. Lung cancer rates were found to be 50% higher than in the general male population of Minnesota and more than two times higher than previously estimated for the Bemidji area of the Indian Health Service (Partin et al. 1996). Also, while the current data confirm the expectation that breast cancer incidence rates are lower among American Indians in Minnesota than in the general population, the differences are much less than in previous studies.

Statistics from the California area office of the Indian Health Service have long been suspected of underreporting due to racial misclassification. At the Intercultural Cancer Council Forum held in Washington, D.C. on March 1, 1999, Dr. E. Sondek, Director of the National Center for Health Statistics, stated that there is suspected an average of 38% underreporting of cancer in American Indians nationwide.

Several published reports have pointed out the limitations of SEER data. Oklahoma is the state with the largest IHS-user population, and the Cherokee Nation of Oklahoma is the largest tribal group in the United States, yet there is no accurate data on cancer incidence and mortality for the Cherokee Nation. Therefore, new efforts are underway to provide technical assistance to the Cherokee Nation to set up an operational cancer registry. Consultants will be drawn from the National Cancer Institute's SEER program staff and investigators, IHS staff, and representatives of the Cherokee Nation.

The Indian Health Service statistical report *Regional Differences in Indian Health 1996* gave the calculated mortality rates for age-adjusted malignant neoplasms for the whole IHS service area as 98.8/100,000, compared to the all–United States rate of 133.1/100,000 (Cobb and Paisano 1997). However, four IHS regional offices—Alaska, Billings (Montana), Bemidji (Minnesota) and Aberdeen (South Dakota)—reported rates higher than the U.S. all-races rates.

The National Center For Health Statistics

Annually, the National Center for Health Statistics conducts the National Health Interview Survey (NHIS). The NHIS provides data on acute illness and injuries, utilization of health services by citizens seventeen or older, and attempts to determine the prevalence of chronic conditions. The survey is conducted in person by census interviewers. Unfortunately, too few Native Americans have been included in this survey format for it to be possible to draw any conclusions about native health issues. While American Indians/Alaska Natives constitute approximately 1% of the U.S. population, the samples have only included 0.006% Native Americans and therefore cannot be regarded as representative.

BARRIERS TO CANCER DETECTION AND TREATMENT

Myths about cancer, distrust and misunderstanding of the health care system, financial barriers, and distance from medical facilities contribute to the late diagnosis of cancer and frequent noncompliance with treatment regimes by American Indian/Alaska Native patients.

Culturally, cancer remains one of the most dreaded diseases in American society, and American Indians and Alaska Natives share this fear. Other sociocultural beliefs about wellness and illness must also be understood if communication barriers are to be overcome.

Theoretically, all federally recognized Native Americans and Alaska Natives have access to health care provided by the federal government through the Indian Health Service. However, on a practical basis this is not the case. Many service units are woefully understaffed and underbudgeted. Rationing of contract health services for procedures and tests that cannot be easily done on the reservation is the norm. For example, screening mammography was not available until the past few years. Even now, the majority of IHS facilities do not have dedicated mammography services, and sporadic use of contracted mobile mammography units is the only form of access.

A major demographic change for American Indians has been relocation to urban areas. The federal program for relocation began in the 1970s with an act of Congress encouraging urban relocation as a way to overcome the abject poverty associated with many reservations. Resources lagged the urbanization process, though; few services have been available, due to inadequate urban Indian clinic program funding. It is estimated that half of all American Indians now live off the reservation in urban areas. As has been seen for other cultural groups and immigrants from foreign countries (Fraumeni et al. 1993), assimilation to the dominant culture has been highly associated with an increase in cancer (Thomas 1979, 103–113). There are currently inadequate resources in most of the major cities to meet the needs of Native Americans who have relocated there.

THE PSYCHOSOCIAL PROBLEMS OF AMERICAN INDIANS/ ALASKA NATIVES WITH CANCER

Within the more socioeconomically advantaged segments of society, there are higher expectations and greater hopes of surviving a diagnosis of cancer than ever before. Access to information has improved, and with this information there has been a major increase in awareness about cancer prevention, early detection, second opinions, and treatment options. Because of these scientific and social changes there has been a steady increase in the number of long-term cancer survivors.

The American Cancer Society estimates that over ten million people in the United States have had cancer at some time in their lives and that over seven million have survived cancer at least five years post-diagnosis (ACS 1999). Survivorship issues have received relatively little attention until recent times, since most of the research efforts have been aimed at determining the success of various treatments rather than looking specifically at survivors and their quality of life (Tross and Holland 1989; Clark and Stovall, 1996). The most complete statistics on Alaska Native cancer survivors have been kept by the SEER data base in the Alaska Tumor Registry, supervised by Dr. Anne Lanier. Those Alaska Natives most likely to be long-term survivors were breast, colorectal, and prostate cancer patients—which are also the cancers with the largest incidence and long-term survivorship in the general population, as well.

Other than data from the Alaska Tumor Registry, there are virtually no firm data available on the numbers of American Indian/Alaska Native cancer survivors. There is even less known about their *quality* of survival.

There have been many taboos related to cancer, and they have made it very difficult for American Indian/Alaska Native cancer survivors to be visible or vocal within their communities. Many patients have been shunned because of the fear cancer invokes. Numerous communities have feared "contamination" by someone returning from the cancer treatment center. The isolation felt by these patients has been painful. Also, many tribal people share the notion that cancer is not a preventable condition.

Fortunately, these misconceptions are slowly being overcome. Making cancer survivors visible and vocal within their communities is a major step toward overcoming the expectation and resignation that once one is diagnosed with cancer, death is likely.

Cancer also evokes guilt feelings. The Indian concept of "being out of balance" is often felt to be causally related to cancer. Patients tend to blame themselves for their disease. Many patients also feel that their cancer stems from genetic predilection or the Creator's will and therefore not due to personal neglect or improper behavior (Weiner 1993).

Several social factors that have been described as contributing to poor adjustment to a cancer diagnosis are commonly found in American Indians/Alaska Natives. Low socioeconomic status, chronic marital or family problems, perceived or actual poor support from others, and absence of affiliation with a meaningful social group can lead to psychiatric problems, alcohol or drug abuse, depression, and chronic anxiety. The development of native cancer support groups is essential to overcome these adjustment problems. No research has been performed yet looking at the behavioral, psychosocial, treatment, and support factors that influence quality of life and survival of American Indian/Alaska Native cancer patients. Research is needed to describe specifically the unmet needs of AI/AN cancer survivors, with a particular focus on their psychosocial adjustment and to identify factors that determine good quality of life during and after treatment.

Many approaches to breaking down the barriers have been tried. Many people within Indian communities are now talking about cancer, teaching patients about the value of screening, educating tribal health boards and leaders, and building partnerships with researchers, state health departments, the Centers for Disease Control, and the National Cancer Institute. Each of these approaches has been valuable and has led to an increase in screening modalities, which ultimately will lead to improvements in survival. The ideal situation will be achieved when we truly know how to teach people to prevent cancer and to restore American Indians and Alaska Natives to their previous state of natural good health.

NATIONAL CONFERENCES ON CANCER IN INDIAN COUNTRY

Because of the paucity of adequate research data and information about cancer in American Indians and Alaska Natives, the Native American Research and Training Center (NARTC) in Tucson, Arizona sponsored a research conference entitled "Cancer in Indian Country" in 1989. The proceedings from this conference were published as a special supplement in the September 1992 issue of the *American Indian Culture and Research Journal.* Among the major outcomes of that conference was the recommendation that cancer survivors be included in future conference activities.

The Network for Cancer Prevention and Control Research among American Indians and Alaska Natives was initiated in 1990 under the auspices of the Special Populations Branch of the National Cancer Institute. The mission of the Network is to improve the health of American Indians and Alaska Native peoples by reducing cancer morbidity and mortality to the lowest possible levels and to improve cancer survival through cancer-control research (see Hampton et al. 1996, 1545–52). The Network has cosponsored two national meetings on "Cancer in Indian Country," in 1991 and 1995, and it sponsored a "Native Women and Cancer" conference held in Tucson in January 1998. A National Strategic Plan for Cancer Prevention and Control to benefit the overall health of American Indians and Alaska Natives has also been published (Burhansstipanov and Dresser 1993).

A second NARTC meeting "Cancer in Indian Country: A National Conference," supported by the National Cancer Institute and the Network for Cancer Control Research among American Indian/Alaska Native Populations was held in Rapid City, South Dakota from September 15–17, 1992. Dr. Judith Kaur led an intertribal panel of cancer survivors, plus the widow of a cancer patient, in talking to the conference attendees about their experiences with cancer and overcoming the barriers of communication. Selected presentations from that meeting were published in vol. 35, no. 4, of *Alaska Medicine*, in 1993. Another outcome of involving cancer survivors in a panel discussion of the image and problems of cancer survivorship was the development of a videotape series on cancer survivors. Initial response to this work has been overwhelmingly positive. The strong impact of the survivors panel also stimulated the IHS Cancer Control Division to provide support for the first native-run cancer support groups and training for support group leaders.

"The Native American Cancer Conference III: Risk Factors, Outreach and Intervention Strategies," was held in Seattle, Washington, June 16-19, 1995. It provided a forum for native community health leaders, clinicians, service providers, researchers, traditional healers, and cancer survivors to exchange information on programs that specifically target American Indians/Alaska Natives as well as Native Hawaiians and American Samoans. Proceedings of that meeting, with details of major cancer prevention and control activities, were published in the journal *Cancer*, as a supplement for the October 1, 1996, issue. The first intertribal support group session was held as part of that conference. Over twenty cancer survivors from fifteen tribes participated in this experience. An impressive litany of isolation, rejection, anger, guilt, and newfound strength was shared. This event reinforced the growing impression that cancer survivors can be mobilized to improve community-based programs to meet the specific needs of native people.

CANCER SUPPORT GROUPS IN AI/AN COMMUNITIES

Until quite recently, as noted, Native American cancer survivors have been "invisible" within their traditional communities. As education of communities and their leaders has increased, cancer survivors have found their voices. One of the most successful organized programs for Native American cancer survivors started in 1990, on the Santo Domingo Pueblo in New Mexico. The group's founder, Ms. Mary Lovato, is a long-term survivor of a bone marrow transplant for treatment of acute leukemia. Ms. Lovato returned to her pueblo commited to breaking the silence surrounding cancer and confronting head-on the social stigmatization that she and her family endured. For example, when she first returned to her pueblo, people would cross the street when they saw her coming, because they were afraid they could catch leukemia from her. With the assistance of one other cancer survivor, she started a cancer support group to offer emotional support, assist others diagnosed with cancer, and educate the pueblo about cancer and cancer survivorship. The group, initially known as "A Gathering of Cancer Support," holds regular meetings at four pueblos. It has also been able to support activities in nine New Mexico pueblos. Members of the support group assist patients by accompanying them to clinic visits and to testing procedures, and providing lay explanations of what the patient can expect. The latter is one of the most valuable services of this program. (A program with a similar support system is the "Native Sisters Program," started by Dr. Linda Burhansstipanov in Los Angeles and Denver [see Burhansstipanov, this volume]).

In 1992, the "People Living Through Cancer, Inc." (PTLC) program, an Albuquerque cancer support organization, adopted and partially funded "A Gathering of Cancer Support Program," and Ms. Lovato became its first director. The program now holds regular training sessions for American Indian and Alaska Natives who wish to set up support networks in their own communities. Since 1995, people from twenty-five tribes have been trained, and often more than fifty people are on a *waiting list* for future training sessions! It is truly a testimony to how one individual can make a difference.

Another example of a successful cancer patient support program is the Southcentral Foundation program, run by Barbara Stillwater. Dr. Stillwater, a member of the Yurok Tribe in Alaska, is the principal investigator and director of the Alaska Native Women's Wellness Project. In 1994–1996, Dr. Stillwater interviewed Alaska Native cancer survivors from each of the major tribes to understand how they had survived the diagnosis of cancer and how they had used their native traditions in their journeys of recovery. The National Cancer Institute funded the Alaska Native Women's Health Project, in which she interviewed over 500 native women about their knowledge and attitudes towards cancer. The result was a project titled "Denaina Tee-ya," which focuses on training community health representatives (CHR's) in developing community support networks and groups for cancer survivors in rural Alaska.

Such programs as the PTLC, Native Sisters, and the Denaina Tee-ya project recognize the importance of spiritual, psychological, social, and physical support services in improving the quality of life of patients being treated for cancer. Empowerment of cancer survivors to lead their communities also increases the opportunities for culturally relevant education about cancer prevention and screening and thereby increases the likelihood that more people in the community will avail themselves of screening services. Knowledge, attitudes, and belief systems must change if behavior is to be influenced positively. These programs show that change *can and will* happen, through committed leaders and the visibility and voices of cancer survivors.

Storytelling is a traditional mode of teaching within native communities. The advocacy of cancer survivors becomes the cornerstone of cancer survivorship. Utilizing videotapes of survivors telling their stories, asking survivors to serve as role models for tribal-run radio and television educational programs, and involving tribal health boards and councils in improving access to screening services are three effective ways to provide culturally meaningful messages about early detection and treatment of cancer and to change gradually the perception of cancer as an unavoidable and uniformly fatal disease.

COMMUNITY EDUCATION AND INTERVENTIONS

From its inception, the Network for Cancer Prevention and Control Research among American Indians and Alaska Native Populations has identified a need for a national resource center for culturally specific and appropriate cancer education and research materials for lay persons, tribal leaders, researchers, and health professionals. That idea came to fruition in 1997, with the dedication of the American Indian/Alaska Native Cancer Information Resources Center and Learning Exchange (Native CIRCLE) in the Mayo Clinic Cancer Center. The long-term objective is to increase culturally sensitive and appropriate research and materials on native communities and to disseminate the knowledge gained from such research to all communities. Ultimately, this will lead to increased prevention, screening, and treatment of cancer and will improve the health of native peoples. Native CIRCLE also serves to connect American Indian and Alaska Native cancer survivors with resources and each other.

The National Cancer Institute is sponsoring studies of the quality of life of cancer survivors as well as collecting data about late complications, such as second malignancies. It is hoped that some of this research will also occur in American Indian/Alaska Native communities, since there is absolutely no current, reputable data about these issues, which face American Indian/Alaska Native cancer survivors.

Because of the new awareness of cancer as a health priority for tribes, the time is ripe for increased efforts at community education and for intervention projects focused on prevention and early detection. Such efforts will ultimately lead to increased numbers of AI/AN cancer survivors. As survivors become more evident and vocal, more people will come forward for screening and education about prevention. Nothing succeeds like success!

SUMMARY

Cancer has not always been a major cause of morbidity and mortality for AI/AN people. Collaborations between the NCI, CDC, and the tribes have raised awareness of cancer as a new health problem and started the development of effective interventions. Much needs to be done to continue this important work. Cancer survivors now exist on every reservation and pueblo and in all major urban Indian communities. Survivors must be mobilized to spread the knowledge that cancer can be treated and cured. Education is the indispensable key but it must be culturally sensitive and relevant. Because of the diversity of the tribes and the heterogeneity of cancer patterns across different tribes and regions of the United States, programs must reflect the priorities and needs of the people they serve.

LITERATURE CITED

American Cancer Society. 1996. *Guidelines at a glance*. Publication 96–50M–no. 2089. Atlanta.

—. 1999. *American Cancer Society facts and figures 1999*. Publication 99–300M–no. 5008.99. Atlanta.

Blot, W. J., A. Lanier, J. F. Fraumeni, Jr. and T. R. Bender. 1975. Cancer mortality among Alaska Natives, 1960–1969. *Journal of the National Cancer Institute* 55(3):547–554.

Burhansstipanov, Linda, and Connie Dresser. 1993. *Native American monograph no. 1: Documentation of the cancer research needs of American Indians and Alaska Natives*. NIH Publication No. 93-3603. Bethesda, MD: National Cancer Institute.

Clark, E. J., and E. L. Stovall. 1996. Advocacy: The cornerstone of cancer survivorship. *Cancer Practice* 4:239–244.

Cobb, Nathaniel, and Roberta E. Paisano, eds. 1997. *Cancer mortality among American Indians and Alaska Natives in the United States: Regional differences in Indian health, 1989–1993.* IHS Pub. No. 97-615–623. Rockville, MD: Indian Health Service.

Creagan, E. T., and J. F. Fraumeni, Jr. 1972. Cancer mortality among American Indians, 1950–1967. *Journal of the National Cancer Institute* 49:959–967.

Dunham, L. J., J. C. Bailar 3d, and G. L. Laqueur. 1973. Histologically diagnosed cancers in 693 Indians of the United States, 1950–1965. *Journal of the National Cancer Institute* 50:1119–1127.

Fraumeni, Joseph F., Jr, Susan S. Devesa, Robert N. Hoover, and Leo J. Kinlen. 1993. Epidemiology of cancer. In *Cancer, principles and practice of Oncology*, ed. Vincent T. De Vita, Jr., Samuel Hellman, and Steven A. Rosenberg, 1504–1505, 4th ed. Philadelphia: Lippincott.

Hampton, James W., Jalna Keala, and Pat H. Luce-Aoelua. 1996. Overview of the National Cancer Institute Networks for cancer control research in Native American populations. *Cancer* 78:1545–1552.

Justice, J. 1989. Bibliography of cancer in Native Americans and Alaska Natives 1800–1988. Tucson: Native American Research and Training Center.

Kaur, Judith S., Marilyn Roubidoux, Jennifer Giroux, Jeffrey Sloan, and Michael Lobell. 1997. Clinical and mammographic correlates of breast disease in Sioux women. *Proceedings of the American Society of Clinical Oncology* 16 Abstract 472:134a.

Lanier, Anne P., Janet Kelly, Bonnie Smith, Claudette Amadon, et al. *Cancer in Alaska Natives: A twenty-five year report 1969–1993.* 1996. Anchorage: Alaska Area Native Health Service, Indian Health Service, Public Health Service, Department of Health and Human Services.

Lee, B. J. 1930. The incidence of cancer among the Indians in the Southwest. *Surgery, Gynecology, and Obstetrics* 50:196–199.

Levin I. 1910. Cancer among the American Indians and its bearing upon the ethnological distribution of the disease. *Z Krebsforsch* 9:422–435.

Mahoney, Martin, and Arthur M. Michalek. 1995. A bibliography of cancer among American Indians and Alaska Natives, 1966–1994. *Alaska Medicine* (April/May/June):63–71.

Partin, Melissa, Jonathan Slater, Jane Korn, et al. 1996. *Cancer incidence among American Indians in Minnesota, 1988–1993.* Minneapolis: Minnesota Department of Public Health.

Reichenbach, D. D. 1967. Autopsy incidence of diseases among Southwestern American Indians. *Archives of Pathology* 84:81–86.

Roubidoux, Marilyn, Judith Salmon Kaur, Jennifer Giroux, Jeffrey Sloan and Michael Lobell. 1998. Mammographic findings and family history risk for breast cancer in Sioux women. *Cancer* 83:1830–1832.

SEER. 1996. *Racial/Ethnic patterns of cancer in the United States 1988–1992.* NIH Pub. No. 96–4104. Bethesda, MD: National Institutes of Health. National Cancer Institute.

Skye, G. E., and J. W. Hampton. 1976. A survey of neoplastic disease in Oklahoma North American aborigines. In *Proceedings of the third international symposium on detection and prevention of cancer*, ed. H. E. Nieburg, 291–296. New York: Dekker.

Thomas, D. B. 1979. *Epidemiologic studies of cancer in minority groups in the western United States.* Bethesda, MD: National Cancer Institute Monograph 53:103–113.

Tross, S., and Jimmie C. Holland. 1989. Psychological sequelae in cancer survivors. In *Handbook of Psycho-oncology*, ed. J. C. Holland and J. H. Rowland, 101–116. New York: Oxford University Press.

Weiner, Diane. 1993. Health beliefs about cancer. *Alaska Medicine* (Oct/Nov/Dec) 4:285–296.

Welty, Thomas, Neva Zephier, Kurt Schweigman, Beverly Blake, and Gary Leonardson. 1993. Cancer risk factors in three Sioux tribes. *Alaska Medicine* (Oct/Nov/Dec) 4:265–274.

Chapter 12

Breast Cancer Screening in Asian and Pacific Islander American Women

Marjorie Kagawa-Singer and Annette E. Maxwell

Breast cancer is the leading site of cancer in women in the United States, including almost all Asian and Pacific Islander American (APA) women (American Cancer Society 1997; Chen and Koh 1997). When breast cancer is found in its early, localized stages, the chances of survival are over 97% (American Cancer Society 1997). Therefore, the United States government report *Healthy People 2000* set the goal of achieving an 80% rate of mammography screening for all women in the United States (U.S. Department of Health and Human Services 1990). APA women have the lowest breast-screening rates of *all* ethnic groups and are far from reaching this goal.

Approximately 180,000 cases of female breast cancer were diagnosed in 1997, with the highest incidence rate in white women, 111.8 new cases per 100,000. The incidence rate for APAs ranged from 28.5 among Korean-American women to 105.6 among Native Hawaiian women (Miller et al. 1996). Aggregated data show APA women have a lower incidence of breast cancer and better general survival rates than white women. The statistics, however, are misleading; they hide the diversity of the APA population. Moreover, the potential cultural reasons for the variances in breast cancer incidence and mortality, and also the psychological and social impacts of the disease on the woman, her family, and community, are virtually unknown. Lack of program and research attention on this population is primarily due to inaccurate, incomplete, and out-of-date statistics. For example, Korean, Filipino, and Native Hawaiian women present later, with more advanced disease, than do their white counterparts, and breast cancer in APAs may appear earlier and more aggressively than in other ethnic groups (Menon et al. 1992).

This chapter presents a brief review of the limited information available on breast cancer screening practices of APA women. We also highlight the intra- and intergroup differences associated with the population of APA women.

DEMOGRAPHICS AND STATISTICS

Since 1965, with the revision of the U. S. immigration law, APAs became the fastest-growing ethnic group in the United States, growing over 100% per decade for the last thirty years. APAs now constitute 2.9% of the total U.S. population (U.S. Department of Commerce 1991), and by the year 2050 this percentage will increase to 10.7% (Lin-Fu 1993). One of the major characteristics of the APA population is its extreme diversity. Over fifty ethnic, cultural, national, and regional groups are grouped in the Asian and Pacific Islander category. The six largest groups in the United States are Chinese (1,645,472), Filipino (1,406,770), Japanese (847,562), Asian Indians (815,447), Korean (798,849), and Vietnamese (614,547). Fifty-one percent are women.

Sampling of the APA population for national databases and research studies is problematic, because of the skewed pattern of residence of APAs in the United States: 56% of APAs live in California, New York, and Hawaii, and 40% of the total APA population live in California alone (U.S. Department of Commerce 1991). The diversity of this population is an even more complex matter than national origin or geographic region of residence. Over 68.2% of the total APA population is foreign born, but each group varies significantly, ranging from approximately 30% of Japanese Americans to over 90% of the Southeast Asians being foreign born (Zane et al. 1994).

Intragroup variation is also significant, since different segments of the population emigrated at different times. They vary by age, social background, education, and reasons for immigration. Moreover, many countries have different subsets of ethnic populations—such as Asian Indians, who have at least fifteen major cultural and language groups from within India alone. Also, the same ethnic group can come from different countries. For example, Chinese immigrants can be from Panama, the Caribbean, or Hong Kong.

Socioeconomic status is one of the major factors influencing health care access and service, and treatment choices. APAs are the only U.S. ethnic population that is overrepresented at both the highest and the lowest ends of the continuum for health indicators of income, education, age, and social status (Tanjasiri et al. 1995).

Income

White Americans have a poverty rate of 6.6%. Poverty rates for APAs range from 6.6% for Japanese Americans to over 70% for some Southeast Asians. APAs have an average household income of $36,784, compared to $31,435 for white Americans, but the poverty and household-income figures are deceiving. Household incomes obscure the facts that APA households may have several wage earners and that sometimes several whole families pool their incomes to support the group. The poverty rate for APAs is 15% nationally, compared to the national average of 11% (United Way 1997). Of APA women over sixty-five years, 14.8% live in poverty and 26% use public assistance (U.S. Bureau of the Census 1993).

Education

The bimodal distribution of APAs on education is hidden by aggregating the groups. Seventy-eight percent of the total U.S. population over the age of twenty-five has a high school education and 21.5% has a college education, compared to 81.8% and 39.1% of APAs overall for high school and college, respectively. Only 26.5% of Laotians and 37.5% of Cambodians have a high school education. Only 2.1% of American women have four or fewer years of elementary school education, compared with 6.2% of APA women (Lin-Fu 1993). Numerous studies indicate that low income and low education constitute major barriers to early cancer detection and screening.

Assimilation/Acculturation

Critical to the understanding of health care decision making by APA women is their degree of assimilation and acculturation into U. S. society. Measurement of these concepts, however, is in a nascent stage. Language use or time in the United States are often used as proxies, but these are gross measures and do not accurately indicate the more subtle influences of the contribution of culture and ethnicity to promoting or maintaining health (Chung and Kagawa-Singer 1994). Studies of migrants indicate that breast cancer rates were 60% higher in APA women than in their native countries (Ziegler et al. 1993). Immigrant women living in the United States for as little as a decade had an 80% higher risk of breast cancer than new immigrants (Menon et al. 1992). For APA women born in the United States, the risk of breast cancer is similar to that for white women.

These migration studies indicate that cultural beliefs and practices affect cancer incidence as well as prevention practices, along with dietary, environmental, and lifestyle factors. The increasing rate of breast cancer in APA women indicates that this disease is affecting growing numbers of APA women and will increase significantly as these women age and acculturate. Effective, culturally based prevention, and early detection programs must be established as quickly as possible.

Age

The median age for APA women is 31.1 years. The median age for *native-born* APA women is 32.5 years, but 15.8 years for foreign-born women. The APA population, however, also has the largest percentage sixty-five years of age and older of all ethnic groups (Kagawa-Singer et al. 1997a). Many of these elderly are poor women with little education or knowledge of the U.S. health care system.

Language

In 1990, one-third of APA 665,605 households were considered "linguistically isolated"—that is, no members over the age of thirteen spoke English "well" or "very well" (U.S. Department of Commerce 1993). Again, the percentage of linguistically isolated elderly varies considerably by APA ethnic group: 55.8% Hmong, 54.9% Cambodian, 54.5% Korean, 53.3% Laotian, 50.0% Vietnamese, 46.5% Chinese, 40.8% Thai, 18.5% Japanese, 17.0% Filipino, and 14.2% Samoan (U.S. Department of Commerce 1993).

BREAST SCREENING PRACTICES

Due to the extreme diversity both within and between ethnic groups, health care behaviors among APA women differ substantially. Yet little is known about the health beliefs and practices for breast screening among APA women. The few national studies that include APA women show that even among the more acculturated, English-speaking women, cancer screening rates are lower than any other ethnic group. Data from the National Health Interview Survey (1987) show that white and black women were more than twice as likely ever to have had a mammogram than women in the Asian/Other category, even after controlling for various demographic characteristics, including education and income (Calle et al. 1993). Data from the 1995 California Behavioral Risk Factor Survey show that 66% of Asian women had received a mammogram in the last two years, compared to 75% of Hispanic, 88% of African-American, and 79% of white women (American Cancer Society 1997). Studies targeting specific Asian-American groups also show low levels of cancer screening rates in Vietnamese (Jenkins et al. 1990; Pham and McPhee 1992; McPhee et al. 1992; McPhee et al. 1996), Chinese (Lovejoy et al. 1989; Chen et al. 1992; Lee et al. 1996), Cambodian (Kelly et al. 1996), Filipino (Maxwell et al. 1997), and Korean (Wismer et al. 1998; Maxwell et al. 1998) women. Screening rates found in these studies are displayed in Table 12.1. Findings from these studies show that Asian women also underutilize clinical breast exams and breast self-examinations.

Only a few studies have examined knowledge, attitudes, and beliefs regarding breast cancer screening in specific Asian ethnic groups. They will be summarized below, followed by a more general discussion of cultural beliefs and practices relevant to selected Asian groups.

Filipino Women

Maxwell and colleagues (1997) interviewed 218 predominantly low-income Filipino women fifty years of age and older. All the women had been born in the Philippines. About half of the interviews were conducted in English and half in Tagalog, the Filipino national language. Based on Anderson et al.'s acculturation scale (1993), which measures language proficiency, language use, and social contact with individuals from native or host cultures, 43% of respondents were classified as traditional (low acculturation), 49% as bicultural (high use of both languages and social contacts with both cultural groups), and 8% as assimilated. Since English is a second language in the Philippines, many Filipino Americans do not have a language barrier, which may have important implications on access to the health care system and information on breast health.

About two-thirds of the women knew the mammography screening guidelines (once a year); 32% of the women correctly identified age and 65% identified family history as risk factors for developing breast cancer. Filipino-American women harbored many different views and misconceptions, including beliefs that breast cancer can be caused by stress (64%), air pollution (48%), doing something morally bad (57%), and hitting or bumping the breast (79%) (only five women believed breast cancer to be contagious). These misconceptions were more common among traditional women than among bicultural or assimilated women. More instructive, however, is that these beliefs did not affect utilization. Therefore, it may be more productive to underscore risk factors, such as age or family history, and to encourage Filipino-American women to screen regularly than to apply scarce resources toward dispelling every misconception regarding breast cancer risk factors.

Barriers to mammography screening appear to be similar to those found in other ethnic groups. Large proportions of women (34–51%) were very concerned about radiation exposure, pain, cost, and the possibility that the mammogram might find cancer. Modesty was a barrier for 18%, who stated that they would be embarrassed to get a mammogram. Filipino-American women have both concrete and attitudinal barriers to mammography utilization.

If a physician recommended a mammogram, 58% of women stated, they would be very likely to get one, but only 57% of the women had received a screening recommendation from a physician. Although 64% of women felt very comfortable requesting a mammogram, 12% did not feel comfortable making such a request.

The strong Roman Catholic influence has been reported to cause many Filipinos to regard illness and suffering as unavoidable in certain circumstances ("It is in God's hands") and to result in a fatalistic attitude towards prevention (Lasky and Martz 1993). Our data appear to support these notions. Thirty-one percent of Filipino-American women in our sample expressed the belief that breast cancer is usually caused by things beyond human control, such as spiritual forces, fate, or predestination; therefore, they felt, they had low control over getting the disease.

It should also be noted that the vast majority of Filipino-American women believed that a mammogram can find breast cancer in its early stages when it is more treatable. This suggests that at least with regard to breast cancer early detection, these women believe in the benefits of early detection.

Korean Women

Maxwell and colleagues (1998) also interviewed 229 predominately low-income Korean-American women fifty years and older. Using Anderson's acculturation scale (1993), 87% were classified as traditional and 13% as bicultural.

Only about half of the sample (49%) knew the American Cancer Society screening guidelines (once a year); about 33% of the women identified age and 59% identified family history as risk factors for developing breast cancer. As in the Filipino sample, misconceptions were common, including the belief that breast cancer can be caused by stress (87%), air pollution (52%), doing something morally bad (38%), and hitting or bumping the breast (27%). These misconceptions were not different between traditional and bicultural women. Also as in the Filipino sample, these misconceptions were not related to mammography screening behavior.

Overall, barriers to breast cancer screening appear to be similar to those found in other ethnic groups (e.g., Bastani et al. 1991; Caplan et al. 1992; Vernon et al. 1992; Fullerton et al. 1996; Kelly et al. 1996; Maxwell et al. 1997). For example, 46–68% of the women were concerned about radiation exposure, pain, cost, the inconvenience of taking time, difficulties reaching the mammography facility, and the possibility of finding breast cancer. Also, 44% were embarrassed about getting a mammogram. Only four Korean women believed breast cancer to be contagious.

Almost 75% of women stated that they were very likely to obtain a mammogram if a physician recommended it. Only 40% of the women had received a screening recommendation from a physician; 44% of women felt very comfortable requesting a mammogram, and 19% felt uncomfortable doing so. These findings, coupled with the fact that the vast majority of the women preferred to receive a mammogram from a Korean health care provider, whom they would regard as the most credible source of health information, underscore the importance of involving Korean health care providers in intervention programs.

As in the Filipino sample, the vast majority of Korean-American women in our sample believed that a mammogram can find breast cancer in its early stages, when it is more treatable.

Vietnamese Women

A number of studies have been conducted with Vietnamese Americans (Jenkins et al. 1990; McPhee et al. 1992; Pham and McPhee 1992; McPhee et al. 1996; Yi 1994). Findings with respect to knowledge of and attitudes regarding breast cancer screening showed that 39% of Vietnamese respondents believed that breast cancer could be caused by poor hygiene, and, unlike the Korean and Filipino women in Maxwell's studies, 29% thought that breast cancer could be contagious. Thirty-seven percent did not know that a breast lump could be a sign of breast cancer, and 55% did not know that family history was a risk factor for breast cancer. The most frequently cited reasons for not receiving breast cancer screening were lack of physician's recommendation, subject's lack of knowledge, embarrassment, cost, and language difficulties (Pham and McPhee 1992). The relatively low acculturation level of these women may be reflected in their responses regarding the etiology of breast cancer and their screening practices.

Chinese Women

The few studies of Chinese Americans have been conducted primarily with low-income women. Data from the National Health Interview survey show that approximately 41% of insured APA women (the majority of whom were Chinese) had never been screened, compared to 30%, 32%, and 43% of white, black, and Hispanic/Latino women, respectively; 75% of uninsured APA women and 40%, 31%, and 60% of white, black, and Hispanic/Latino women, respectively had not been screened (Kagawa-Singer et al. 1997a). Other studies indicate screening rates that range from 12% (Lovejoy et al. 1989) to 70% (Lee et al. 1996). Higher acculturation, lower age, and higher socioeconomic status were significantly associated with increased screening rates (Lovejoy et al. 1989; Chen et al. 1992; Lu 1995; Lee et al. 1996).

CULTURAL BELIEFS AND PRACTICES

The screening studies reported thus far identify barriers to screening that are similar to those found among other ethnic groups; they include lack of physician referrals, availability, accessibility, acceptability, risks perceived as greater than benefits, structural issues, lack of knowledge, cost or lack of insurance, and fear of cancer. Few studies, however, attempt to identify specific cultural beliefs and practices that may discourage screening behavior, such as varying concepts of health and causes of cancer, concepts regarding the body and the value of the breasts, language issues, intragroup diversity, and conceptualizations of the "problem" caused by breast cancer, such as death, disability, or disfigurement (McElroy and Townsend 1989; Kagawa-Singer et al. 1997b). Importantly, no efforts have been made to identify and use health-*promoting* cultural beliefs and practices, such as attitudes toward preventive health practices and role responsibilities to family, to encourage screening practices.

Only one paper describes in any depth an ethnographic approach to cultural perspectives on breast screening. Mo (1992) has reported on the cultural beliefs and practices of Chinese-speaking women in the San Francisco area. Particular beliefs and values for women in Chinese culture may have profound influences on the use of breast screening practices. Only six of sixty-two new immigrant Chinese speaking women thought it was important to have regular medical checkups. The reluctance seemed to be due to the inconvenience and cost of seeing a physician. These women also believed, however, that the female organs do not function, or cease to function, if they are not used in procreation (unmarried or elderly women); therefore, examination of the breast, uterus, ovaries, and cervix is unnecessary. Moreover, for an unmarried woman to have such examinations would be an admission she was a sexual being and able to procreate—an idea of sexual activity that would be both immodest and repugnant. Mo's study emphasizes the need to conduct with APA women cultural assessments that include the social and cultural context of the women interviewed regarding beliefs about health, sexuality, and fertility.

Levin et al. (1997) report on a study of mobile mammography use by low-income women. Asian-American women availed themselves of the screening at a significantly higher rate than white, African-American, or Hispanic women. Even though the low-cost mobile van eliminated the structural barriers to mammography, 43% (thirty-three of seventy-six) of the women who declined the service gave "miscellaneous reasons" for not obtaining a breast examination and mammogram, such as not feeling well, did not want to leave friends, had to leave, bad experience with previous mammogram, and a belief that the individual cannot interfere with God's will. Women also gave managed-care insurance coverage, lack of physician referral, advanced age, and life not being worth living as other reasons. Additional studies are needed to tease out the cultural factors that may underlie the general "excuses" given by APA and other ethnic women for not utilizing breast screening services.

In an ethnographic study of acculturated Chinese, Japanese, and Filipino American women living in Los Angeles, Ito (1982) found significant group differences in attitudes toward health and illness. The Chinese-American women seemed to view health skeptically: illness was problematic, and health was not certain. Despite appearances and good medical care and health habits, these women felt that one never knew when sudden death, severe illness, or psychological problems might develop. Attempts to maintain good physical health focused on particular attention to food and cooking styles, with emphasis on Chinese cooking being "better for you" and "healthier." Unexpected maladies caused constant concern and worry.

The Japanese-American women interviewed saw health as a matter of will. Dwelling on oneself or even preventive monitoring was self-indulgent and reprehensible: "If you think about getting sick, you will." Prevention took the form of ignoring symptoms and performing daily duties and work to keep from feeling bad. Correct attitude and thinking were powerful controls over one's state of health.

Filipino women seemed to consider health as a moral statement about the correct fulfillment of social, and in particular kin, obligations. Religious devotion, faith in God and His will was a *leitmotif* in these Filipino-American lives. In contrast to Japanese Americans, for Filipino Americans the important relationship for health maintenance and illness prevention was that between body and soul, rather than between body and mind (Ito et al. 1997).

Kagawa-Singer and colleagues (1997b) found that differences in cultural concepts of the body and self between mainstream white women and Japanese- and Chinese-American women with breast cancer may create barriers to optimal cancer care. Three possible explanations influence their respective use of breast screening services, related to the cultural values and beliefs that underlie these behaviors. First, in Western society the duality of mind and body is hierarchical, with intellect over emotions and the soma. In the West, somatic distress is considered to be a secondary communication of primary psychological distress (Simon and Von Korff 1991; Kawanishi 1992) and, most critically, is considered best understood by translating it into its underlying psychological etiology. In the

Confucian, Buddhist, and Hindu traditions, feelings and intuition have a higher value than words. Intellect and psychological or somatic distress are synonymous. For those who hold Eastern perspectives, somatic presentation of complaints is not due to a lack of vocabulary or sophistication in understanding the "psychological" processes going on but to conceptual differences in the primacy of the body as the *appropriate* symbolic vehicle of communication of both emotional and physical distress (Eisenberg 1977; Ots 1990). It is *understood* that this integrative dysfunction is brought on by emotional/environmental imbalances. Separating mind and body into separate disciplinary domains is inconceivable in the Asian worldview. Such a view may reduce the effectiveness of current messages promoting breast cancer screening. Most health education messages stress cancer as the threat and responsibility to one's *self* as the motivating factor for early detection. If the mind/body connection is as interrelated for APAs as the literature indicates, thinking about cancer or even saying the words potentially can cause the cancer (Ito 1982; Carrese and Rhodes 1995; see also Weiner, this volume), and focusing on the self as opposed to one's role in the family is reprehensible.

The role of the woman is also intertwined with the concept of in Japanese, *shikataganai*, "such is the way things happen"—in Chinese, *ming chung chu ting*, or "misfortune is predestined." In this philosophy, though having cancer is personally difficult, the traditional role of the woman in these two Asian cultures is to maintain harmony in their families *in spite of their own needs*, not focusing upon themselves. Thus, focusing their energies on the needs of others, they may not choose preventive services that would reduce resources for their loved ones (especially low-income women), reflecting the socially valued practice of self-sacrifice.

The emotional cost/benefit relationship may also be a factor. In Far Eastern cultures, self-sufficiency is highly valued (Kagawa-Singer 1988). To focus on oneself is viewed as selfish and disrespectful, and it results in loss of face. "Face" is a pivotal value in APA culture. This concept means more than "self-respect" or individual "dignity," as conceived in Western culture. In APA culture, individual needs are subsumed by the welfare of the group; one strives to maintain "face" because it embraces the integrity of one's entire family and even one's community (Kagawa-Singer and Chung 1994; Zane et al. 1994).

Last, in Asian cultures overall, a woman is expected to sacrifice her own sense of well-being for the welfare of her family, to suffer in silence, and to endure psychological distress (Lock 1983). Using breast screening practices for her own welfare, when it costs money and time, and especially if she has no symptoms, may be perceived as selfish—a perception that may constitute a significant barrier to early detection.

COMMUNICATION WITH PHYSICIANS

Differences in patient and physician expectations of communication styles may also create barriers to early detection and screening practices (Wellisch et al. 1999). The expected, standard American mode of communication between provider and patient is direct and open for both participants (Nilchaikovit et al. 1993). In cancer care, patients are expected and encouraged to verbalize their concerns and make them known in a direct fashion. In Asian cultures, the mode of polite communication, especially between practitioner and patient, is one of deference and indirectness (Hsu et al. 1985; Mink and Nihira 1987). Thus, even if more traditional APA women feel they were asking their physicians questions, the *manner* in which they do so may be confusing or unclear for Euro-American or American-trained practitioners. On the other hand, the Asian expectation may be that the physician will be paternalistic (Ishiwata and Sakai 1994). In such a relationship, the woman would expect the physician to anticipate her needs and provide for them—for example, ordering the mammogram without her having to ask. If the physician does not address an area of the patient's concern, even a nonverbalized one, she may feel it unwarranted to ask (since it appears not to be significant enough for the doctor to address) and impolite for her to raise the issue (since it would appear to criticize the doctor's knowledge).

Meredith (1994) found that Asian patients report statistically significantly greater difficulty in communicating with their physicians than do African-American, European-American, and Hispanic patients. No studies, however, indicate the nature of the communication difficulties. More definitive information on the interactions with the physicians by Asian-American patients is required to identify the culturally framed presentation of symptoms of physical and emotional distress and to design interventions that would provide information about breast cancer and screening practices in a more culturally effective manner, so as to increase utilization.

SUCCESSFUL SCREENING PROGRAMS

Screening programs that have proven successful in APA communities have demonstrated the same strategies used by programs in other "hard to reach" populations. *Culturally congruent and competent* practices, coupled with the public health model of participatory program development, encompass these overlapping strategies. These entail five basic structural elements of service delivery: that they be accessible, affordable, acceptable, appropriate, and accountable within a culturally competent institutional environment (Higgenbotham 1984; Cross et al. 1989; Orlandi et al. 1992)

Accessibility requires that an agency have the language capability necessary for serving different populations, that it have staff who are bilingual and bicultural. Accessibility also requires that the agency be accessible at the level of literacy of the population, in the language required. This also means that literature and videos must be language and literacy-level appropriate and that the message be provided in the medium most effective for the learning needs of the group, such as storytelling versus lecturing. The services themselves must also be convenient; sites where all services can be provided at one location and at one time appear to have the greatest success for women of all ethnic groups. For low-acculturated women, multiservice centers are also highly effective, because attendance is not specific to one disorder, preserving her privacy in the community. Others in the community cannot as easily know the specific service for which she is utilizing the center.

Screening services must also be affordable. Low-cost cancer screening services are essential, for many APA women are uninsured or underinsured—especially for prevention and screening services. It is often reported that APA women are not prevention oriented (see McPhee et al. 1996). This concept would be contrary to traditional APA health constructs of balance in all aspects of one's life—physical, mental, emotional, and spiritual—a balance that requires attention to one's emotional state, level of exercise, emotional attitude, and diet. Perhaps the difference is due to the exigencies of life in the United Stated refugee population, differing concepts of how cancers start and work in the body, and varying realizations that something can be done about it. Cultural issues for APA women of self-sacrifice for the family, especially in light of the needs of the family, must also be assessed for their influence on screening behaviors.

The acceptability of the program to the group requires that credible community leaders endorse the program and be involved in developing it from the inception of the idea. Credible community teachers of the material must also be available (Bandura 1986). In breast screening programs, these individuals are often women of and in the community who are trained and paid as peer educators.

The format and presentation must also be appropriate. Often the design of the intervention has been predetermined and the message is in a format that is not appropriate, for instance asking direct questions about sensitive areas rather than taking a more appropriate and perhaps time-consuming indirect route (Mo 1992). The format for less-educated women tends to be small-group settings (large enough to promote discussion but small enough to remain intimate), often in culturally sanctioned locations (e.g., community halls or homes). The message, as noted earlier, is often most successful when it addresses the woman's chief responsibility: the well-being of her family (Sabogal et al. 1996). The American Cancer Society has a poster that addresses Asian-American women directly (its message is written in thirteen Asian languages) and the theme is "healthy mothers—healthy families."

The last required element is accountability. Too often public health programs are implemented by outside agencies, whose grants require short start-up timelines. This, by definition, means that the preparatory work may be superficial and that the projects are time limited and often narrowly focused. Screening programs are often funded for screening only; follow-up for diagnostic work or treatment is not part of the program. Who, then, is accountable for the program and for care along the entire continuum for the women who participate? What steps have been taken to support these women after funding ends? If there are concerns or complaints, what recourse do the women or participating community agency have? Community agencies have become much more sophisticated in their participation in such programs, and they require that such questions be answered before they endorse them.

Program objectives are also held up to scrutiny. For example, APA groups are often left out of the planning for outreach programs to "minority" or "hard to reach" populations. This brings us back to the lack of accurate data: it is often assumed that this is not a population in need. The other side of the coin also occurs, however. Once agencies recognize that the APA population has needs, program developers try to serve specific populations and then face the issue of small numbers and low generalizability. Program developers, researchers, and funding sources must begin to recognize the contribution of culturally competent practice.

IMPLICATIONS AND RECOMMENDATIONS

APA women face two categories of problems that must be simultaneously addressed to increase screening utilization (Kagawa-Singer 1997). The first is structural—such generic problems as accessible, affordable, and logistically convenient health services. These problems pose significant barriers to APA women of low acculturation. Specific structural factors that would facilitate use of services for APA women of limited acculturation are (1) availability of providers of the same ethnicity; (2) bicultural and bilingual staff; (3) respectful communication styles by staff; (4) health education materials in the appropriate language and at the correct literacy level; (5) affordability of services; and (6) multiservice centers to reduce the need for multiple appointments in different geographic locations or for multiple, uncoordinated visits (Ho 1989).

The second category comprises such conceptual issues as knowledge about the causes of cancer, understanding that cancer can be cured, specific attitudes, beliefs and values of particular ethnic groups toward cancer in general and specifically toward preventive health care practices, and use of screening modalities (Ho 1989).

The assumptions underlying the structures of most current screening programs reflect the white, mainstream values of individualism, autonomy, and assertiveness for individual health needs. These values promote modes of communication that are antithetical to the APA rules of interpersonal interactions (Leininger 1991). The relationship in the mainstream paradigm is between the individual and institution as a resource. Successful ethnic-specific programs are congruent with cultural values, provide more personalized services fostering trust between the provider and the woman, and are bilingual and bicultural. In these programs a health-promotion approach, with an educational focus, is used, rather than an emotional appeal to individual needs. Effective delivery also supports the value of women's roles in the family and employs outreach workers who are respected women from the community.

Education of health practitioners is essential. Multiple studies have indicated that the single most effective stimulus for mammography is a referral from a physician, yet physicians seeing APA women, and especially older women of all ethnic groups, seem to suffer from the misconception that breast cancer is not a risk or that aggressive, proactive measures are not indicated (Caplan et al. 1992; O'Malley et al. 1997). This myth must be dispelled.

Alternative or complementary health activities and practitioners are widely used in many of the APA groups. Western biomedical clinicians must determine if these practices are helpful, neutral, or maladaptive. If the practice or practitioner is helpful or neutral, these practices can be supported. Such support and integration would indicate respect for cultural beliefs. Mainstream practitioners might also learn other effective ways to promote positive health practices. If a practice is harmful, practitioners must work with the community and families to help them understand how it may be counterproductive.

All cultures attempt to maintain the health and welfare of its members, but the ways in which they achieve this end are often culturally specific, due to differing worldviews, concepts of health, and roles of women. Other mediating factors must also be addressed when developing programs for APA women, such as language ability, age, socioeconomic status, and emotional and social resources. By addressing the culture-general as well as culture-specific needs and drawing on the richness of the natural cultural-support systems and integrating them with Western therapeutic techniques, screening and early detection efforts can decrease the morbidity and mortality of APA women from breast cancer.

LITERATURE CITED

American Cancer Society. 1997. *California cancer facts and figures.* Atlanta.

Anderson, J., M. Moeschberger, M. S. Chen, Jr., P. Kunn, M. E. Wewers, and R. Guthrie. 1993. An acculturation scale for Southeast Asians. *Social Psychiatry, Psychiatric Epidemiology* 28:134–141.

Bandura, A. 1986. *Social foundations of thought and action: A social cognitive theory.* Engelwood Cliffs, NJ: Prentice-Hall.

Bastani, R., A. C. Marcus, and A. Hollatz-Brown. 1991. Screening mammography rates and barriers to use: A Los Angeles County survey. *Preventive Medicine* 20:350–363.

Berry, J. W., and U. Kim. 1988. Acculturation and mental health. In *Health and cross-cultural psychology: toward applications,* ed. P. R. Dasen, J. W. Berry, and N. Satorius, 207–236. Newbury Park, CA: Sage.

Calle, E. E., W. D. Flanders, M. J. Thun, and L. M. Martin. 1993. Demographic predictors of mammography and Pap smear screening in U.S. women. *American Journal of Public Health* 83:53–60.

Caplan, L. S., B. L. Wells, and S. Haynes. 1992. Breast cancer screening among older racial/ethnic minorities and whites: Barriers to early detection. *Journal of Gerontology* 47: 101–110.

Carrese, J. A., and L. A. Rhodes. 1995. Western bioethics on the Navajo reservation: Benefit or harm? *Journal of the American Medical Association* 274(10):826–829.

Chen, A., R. Lew, V. Thai, K. L. Ko, L. Okahara, S. Hirota, S. Chan, W. F. Wong, G. Saika, L. F. Folkers, and B. Marquez. 1992. Behavioral risk factor survey of Chinese—California, 1989. *MMWR* 41:266–270.

Chen, M., and H. Koh. 1997. The need for cancer prevention and control among Asian Americans and Pacific Islanders. *Asian American and Pacific Islander Journal of Health* 5(1):3–6.

Chung, R-Y. C., and Kagawa-Singer, M. 1994. Predictors of psychological distress among Southeast Asian refugees. *Social Science and Medicine* 36(5):631–639.

Cross, T. L., B. J. Bazron, K. W. Dennis, and M. R. Isaacs. 1989. *Towards a culturally competent system of care: A monograph on effective services for minority children who are severely emotionally disturbed*. Washington, DC: Child and Adolescent Service System Program Technical Assistance Center, Georgetown University Child Development Center.

Eisenberg, L. 1977. Disease and illness. *Culture, Medicine and Psychiatry* 1(9):9–23.

Fullerton, J. T., D. Kritz-Silverstein, G. R. Sadler, and E. Barrett-Connor. 1996. Mammography usage in a community-based sample of older women. *Annals of Behavioral Medicine* 18:67–72.

Higgenbotham, H. N. 1984. *Third world challenge to psychiatry*. Honolulu: East-West Center, University of Hawaii Press.

Ho, M. K. 1989. Applying family therapy theories to Asian/Pacific Americans. Annual program meetings of the Council on Social Work Education (1987, St. Louis, Missouri). *Contemporary Family Therapy: An International Journal* 11(1):61–70.

Hsu, J., W. S. Tseng, G. Ashton, J. McDermott, and W. Char. 1985. Family interaction patterns among Japanese American and Caucasian families in Hawaii. *Journal of Psychiatry* 142(5):477–581.

Ishiwata, R., and A. Sakai. 1994. The physician-patient relationship and medical ethics in Japan. *Cambridge Quarterly of Health Care Ethics* 3:60–66.

Ito, K. L. 1982. *NIMH final report: Health care alternatives of Asian American women*.

Ito, K. L., R-Y. C. Chung, and M. Kagawa-Singer. 1997. Asian/Pacific American women: Health care issues of a multicultural group. In *Women's Health: Complexities and Differences*, ed. Sheryl Burt Ruzek, Virginia Olesen, and Adele E. Clarke, 300–328. Columbus: Ohio State University Press.

Jenkins, C. N. H., S. J. McPhee, J. A Bird, and N. T. Bonilla. 1990. Cancer risks and prevention practices among Vietnamese refugees. *Western Journal of Medicine* 153:34–39.

Kagawa-Singer, M. 1988. Bamboo and Oak: Differences in the adaptation to cancer between Japanese-American and Anglo-American patients. Ph.D. dissertation, University of California, Los Angeles.

—. 1997. Issues affecting Asian American American Women. *Contemporary Issues in Breast Cancer*, ed. K. Hassey Dow, 229–242. Boston: Jones and Bartlett.

Kagawa-Singer, M., and R. Chung. 1994. A paradigm for culturally based care for minority populations. *Journal of Community Psychology* 22(2):192–208.

Kagawa-Singer M., N. Hikoyeda, and S. P. Tanjsiri. 1997a. Health issues for elderly Asian Pacific Islanders. In *Minorities, Aging and Health*, ed. K. Markides and M. Miranda, 149–180. Thousand Oaks, CA: Sage.

Kagawa-Singer, M., D. K. Wellisch, and R. Durvasula. 1997b. Impact of breast cancer on Asian American and Anglo American Women. *Culture, Medicine and Psychiatry* 21:449–480.

Kawanishi, Y. 1992. Somatization of Asians: An artifact of Western medicalization. *Transcultural Psychiatric Research Review* 29:5–36.

Kelly, A. W., M. Chacori, P. C. Wollan, M. A. Trapp, A. L. Weaver, P. A. Barrier, W. B. Franz, and T. E. Kottke. 1996. A program to increase breast and cervical cancer screening for Cambodian women in a Midwestern community. *Mayo Clinic Proceedings* 71:437–444.

Lasky, E. M., and C. H. Martz. 1993. The Asian/Pacific Islander population in the US: Cultural perspectives and their relationship to cancer prevention and early detection.

In *Cancer Prevention in Minority Populations*, ed. M. Frank-Stromborg and S. Olsen, 80–112. St. Louis: Mosby.

Lee, M., F. Lee, S. Stewart. 1996. Pathways to early breast and cervical detection for Chinese American women. *Health Education Quarterly* 23(Supplement):S76–S88.

Leininger, M. 1991. Culture care diversity and universality: A theory of Nursing. New York: National League for Nursing Press. Pub. No. 15–2402. *Nursing and Health Care* 6(4):209–212.

Levin, J. R., S. H. Hirsch, R. Bastani, P. A. Ganz, M. L. Lovett, D. Reuben. 1997. Acceptability of mobile mammography among community-dwelling seniors. *Journal of the American Geriatrics Society* 45:1365–1375.

Lin-Fu, J. S. 1993. Asian and Pacific Islanders: An overview of demographic characteristics and health care issues. *Asian American and Pacific Islander Journal of Health* 1(1):20–36.

Lock, M. 1983. Licorice in leviathan: The medicalization of care for the Japanese elderly. *Culture, Medicine and Psychiatry* 8(2):121–139.

Lovejoy, N. C., C. Jenkins, T. Wu, S. Shankland, and C. Wilson. 1989. Developing a breast cancer screening program for Chinese-American women. *Oncology Nursing Forum* 16:181–187.

Lu, J. Z. 1995. Variables associated with breast self-examination among Chinese women. *Cancer Nursing* 18(1):29–34.

Maxwell, A. E., R. Bastani, and U. S. Warda. 1997. Breast cancer screening and related attitudes among Filipino-American women. *Cancer Epidemiology, Biomarkers and Prevention* 6:719–726.

—. 1998. Mammography utilization and related attitudes among Korean-American women. *Women and Health* 27:89–107.

McElroy, A. and P. K. Townsend. 1989. *Medical Anthropology*. Boulder, CO: Westview.

McPhee S. J., J. A. Bird, N. T. Ha, C. Jenkins, D. Fordham, and B. Le. 1996. Pathways to early cancer detection for Vietnamese women: Suc khoe la vang! (health is gold). *Health Education Quarterly* 23(Supplement):S60–S75.

McPhee, S. J., C. N. H. Jenkins, S. Hung, K. P. Nguyen, N. T. Ha, and D. C. Fordham. 1992. Behavioral Risk Factor Survey of Vietnamese—California, 1991. *Morbidity and Mortality Weekly Report*. U.S. Department of Health and Human Services, Public Health Service 41(5).

Menon, M., C. H. The, and C. L. Chua. 1992. Clinical and social problems in young women with breast carcinoma. *Australian and New Zealand Journal of Surgery* 62(5):364–367.

Meredith, L. 1994. Health of Asians and Pacific Islanders in the medical outcomes study. UCLA/MEDTEP Outcomes Research Center for Asians and Pacific Islanders, unpublished project report.

Miller, B. A., L. N. Kolonel, L. Bernstein, J. L. Young, Jr., G. M. Swanson, D. West, C. R. Key, J. M. Liff, C. S. Glover, G. A. Alexander, et al., eds. 1996. Racial/ethnic patterns of cancer in the United States 1988–1992. NIH Pub. No. 96-4104. Bethesda, MD: National Cancer Institute.

Mink, I. T., and K. Nihira. 1987. Direction of effects: Family life styles and behavior of TMR children. *American Journal of Mental Deficiency* 92 (1):57–64.

Mo, B. 1992. Modesty, sexuality, and breast health in Chinese-American women. In Crosscultural medicine: A decade later [special issue]. *Western Journal of Medicine* 157:260–264.

Morris, C. R., and W. E. Wright. 1996. *Breast cancer in California*. Sacramento: Cancer Surveillance Section, Department of Health Services, State of California.

Nilchaikovit, T. N., J. M. Hill, and J. C. Holland. 1993. The effects of culture on illness behavior and medical care: Asian and American differences. *General Hospital Psychiatry* 15:41–50.

O'Malley, A. S., J. Madelblatt, K. Gold, K. A. Cagney, and J. Kerner. 1997. Continuity of care and the use of breast and cervical cancer screening services in a multiethnic community. *Archives of Internal Medicine* 157:1462–1740.

Orlandi, M. A., R. Weston, and L. Epstein. 1992. *Cultural competence for evaluators.* DHHS Publication (ADM)92–1884. Rockville, MD: U.S. Department of Health and Human Services, Office of Substance Abuse Prevention, Division of Community Prevention and Training.

Ots, T. 1990. The angry liver, the anxious heart and the melancholy spleen. *Culture, Medicine and Psychiatry* 14:21–58.

Pham, C. T., and S. J. McPhee. 1992. Knowledge, attitudes, and practices of breast and cervical cancer screening among Vietnamese women. *Journal of Cancer Education* 7:305–310.

Sabogal, F., R. Otero-Sabogal, R. J. Pasick, C. N. H. Jenkins, and E. J. P. Perez-Stable. 1996. Printed health education materials for diverse communities: Suggestions learned from the field. *Health Education Quarterly* 23(supplement):S123–S141.

Simon, G. E., and M. Von Korff. 1991. Somatization and psychiatric disorder in the NIMH epidemiologic catchment area study. *American Journal of Psychiatry* 148(11):1494–1500.

Tanjasiri, S. P., S. P. Wallace, and K. Shibata. 1995. Picture imperfect: Hidden problems among Asian Pacific Islander elderly. *Gerontologist* 35(6):753–760.

United Way of Greater Los Angeles. 1997. *Asian Pacific Profiles: Los Angeles County.* Los Angeles: United Way of Greater Los Angeles.

U.S. Bureau of the Census. 1993. Money income of households, families, and persons in the United States: 1992. *Current Population Reports*, Series P60-184. Washington, DC: Government Printing Office.

U.S. Department of Commerce. 1991. *Census Bureau releases 1990 census counts on specific racial groups*, CB 91-215. Washington, DC: Bureau of the Census.

—. 1993. *We the Americans: Pacific Islanders.* Economics and Statistics Administration. Washington, DC: Bureau of the Census.

U.S. Department of Health and Human Services. 1990. *Healthy People 2000.* Washington, DC: Government Printing Office.

Vernon, S. W., V. G. Vogel, S. Halabi, G. L. Jackson, R. O. Lundy, and G. N. Peters. 1992. Breast cancer screening behaviors and attitudes in three racial/ethnic groups. *Cancer* 69:165–174.

Wellisch, D. K., M. Kagawa-Singer, S. Reid, Y-J. Lin, S. Nishikawa, and M. Wellisch. 1999. An exploratory study of social support: A cross-cultural comparison of Chinese, Japanese, and Anglo-American breast cancer patients. *Psycho-Oncology* 8:207-219.

Wismer, B. A., J. M. Moskowitz, A. M. Chen, S. H. Kang, T. E. Novotny, R. Lew, and I. B. Tager. 1998. Mammography and clinical breast examination among Korean American women in two California counties. *Preventive Medicine:* 27:144–151.

Yi, J. K. 1994. Breast cancer screening practices by Vietnamese women. *Journal of Women's Health* 3:205–213.

Zane, N. W. S., D. T. Takeuchi, and K. N. J. Young. 1994. *Confronting critical health issues of Asian and Pacific Islander Americans.* Thousand Oaks, CA: Sage.

Ziegler, R. G., R. N. Hoover, M. C. Pike, A. Hildesheim, A. M Nomura, D. W. West, A. H. Wu-Williams, et al. 1993. Migration patterns and breast cancer risk in Asian-American women. *Journal of the National Cancer Institute* 85(22):1819–1827.

Table 12.1
Studies of Breast Cancer Screening Rates of Asian-American Women

Reference	Study methodology	Screening rates (note: White women 1989-90: 73% ever had a mammogram)
McPhee et al. 1992	Telephone interviews in Vietnamese with 1,011 Vietnamese residing in California (out of a random sample of 1,705; response rate 59%).	Among women 40+ (N=195), 52% ever had a mammogram.
McPhee et al. 1996	Face-to-face interviews in Vietnamese with 645 women 18+ in San Francisco and Sacramento (out of 6,188 households contacted; response rate approximately 79%).	Among women 40+ (N=276), 50% ever had a mammogram. Among women 50+ (N=132), 48% ever had a mammogram.
Yi 1994	Telephone interviews in Vietnamese (86%) or English (14%) with 141 Vietnamese women ages 18-65 (out of 233 eligible women; response rate 60%).	50% ever had a CBE and 87% had had a CBE during the past 12 months. Among women 40+ (N=54), 65% ever had a mammogram.
Chen et al. 1992	Face-to-face interviews in Cantonese with 296 Chinese living in Oakland (out of a random sample of 359; response rate 82%).	Among women 40+(N=100), 32% ever had a mammogram and 25% ever did BSE.
Lee et al. 1996	Telephone interviews in English, Mandarin and Cantonese with 450 Chinese-American women living in San Francisco.	Among women 40+(N=540), 70% ever had a mammogram. Among women 50+ (N=308), 55% had a mammogram in the past year.
Kelly et al. 1996	Medical record reviews of Cambodian women 50+ (N=57), who had received health care between 1985 and 1992 in at least one of three medical institutions in Olmsted County, Minnesota	In a 12 months period, 12% had received a mammogram and 21% had received a CBE.
Maxwell et al. 1997	Face-to-face interviews (50% English, 50% Tagalog) with a convenience sample of 218 Filipino women 50+ residing in Los Angeles.	66% ever had a mammogram, 54% had a mammogram in the past 2 years, 34% have CBE yearly, 69% do BSE monthly or more frequently.
Maxwell et al. 1998	Face-to-face interviews in Korean with a convenience sample of 229 Korean women 50+ residing in Los Angeles.	49% ever had a mammogram, 36% had a mammogram in the past 2 years, 22% have CBE yearly, 32% do BSE monthly or more frequently.
Wismer et al. 1998	Population based telephone survey with Korean-American adults in Alameda and Santa Clara counties, California (424 women 50+)	Among women 50+, 34% had a mammogram in the past 2 years, 32% had CBE in the past 2 years.
Kagawa-Singer et al. 1997a	Review of medical records of low income women in community based ethnic clinics: Chinese N=248, Korean N=229, Thai N = 115, Vietnamese N=33	Ever had a mammogram: Chinese, 54.8%, Korean 32,3%, Thai 25.2% and Vietnamese, 24.2% CBE/BSE: C = 65.7, K = 11.8, Thai = 56.5, V = 66.7

Part III

New Strategies for Cancer Research

Chapter 13

Developing Culturally Competent Community-Based Interventions

Linda Burhansstipanov

INTRODUCTION

This chapter briefly highlights selected issues that need to be addressed to increase the likelihood of developing and implementing culturally competent interventions in American Indian and Alaska Native communities. Many of the same issues are relevant to other cultures, but the interventions to address them must be competent for the specific and intended population. The majority of community-based projects are required to collect local data to *identify barriers* to participation in cancer prevention and control programs. However, the emphasis needs to be refocused toward developing and implementing culturally competent interventions that can effectively address those barriers. Most community-based organization (CBO) leaders can tell a researcher about the barriers in the community. In working with diverse communities, our Native Women's Wellness through Awareness (NAWWA) staff have concluded that survey data typically identify the poverty-related barriers (Burhansstipanov et al. 1998a). These are very real and do need to be addressed; however, after addressing the poverty-related barriers we have found little or no change in community participation in early detection programs. In the face of this situation, we have coordinated focus groups with community leaders to determine what was really happening.

To illustrate briefly, during the NAWWA Project (Denver and Los Angeles), trained staff administered survey instruments to the participants. Survey data indicated that elder American Indian women needed transportation and child care (many care for their grandchildren). These two factors, both poverty related, were clearly the most profound barriers affecting participation in early detection programs. During a focus group we learned that the poverty-related barriers were "easier" for respondents to "answer" but that the actual barriers to screening were sociocultural. But sociocultural responses would have been "harder" and take longer for the respondent to explain; therefore, it was "easier" to just indicate poverty barriers. This is not to imply that transportation barriers are not real—they are. It indicates that even when transportation barriers are addressed, the researcher/service provider must address other barriers, which are less likely to appear on survey findings.

OBJECTIVE 1: DISTINGUISH AMONG CULTURALLY "SENSITIVE," "RELEVANT," APPROPRIATE," "ACCEPTABLE," AND "COMPETENT"

Prior to delving into cultural interventions, the reader needs a basic set of definitions of terms used in different manners throughout this chapter. These include "culturally appropriate," "relevant," "competent," "sensitive," and "acceptable" cancer interventions, services, or programs (see Table 13.1). There is much confusion between these terms, but rather than haggle about the terminology, the "concepts" or ideas behind the terms are more important than the definitions. For the purposes of the discussion in this chapter, these terms can be briefly described. "Culturally sensitive" means that the strategy is respectful to the participating culture, community, and leaders. A culturally sensitive recruitment may include working with the traditional Indian healer in a *leadership* role during a cancer pain-management project. "Culturally appropriate" means that a strategy is presented in language or phrasing that accurately communicates the meaning to the participant, or a literacy level that is designed for the average reading level of the intended population. "Culturally relevant" means that the project, strategy, or informational item is specifically targeted to the participant and that the participant would perceive it as relevant to his or her health. "Culturally competent" means that the program/project is appropriate, sensitive, relevant, and acceptable to the participant.

Table 13.1 "Cultural" Definitions	
• *sensitive*—	respectful of the specific culture's beliefs, practices, and so on
• *relevant*—	specifically targeted to a definite culture
• *appropriate*—	respectful, relevant to specific culture and literacy issues
• *acceptable*—	not appropriate, but due to some factor, is "permissible" to be used/implemented within the targeted community
• *competent*—	incorporates culturally sensitive, relevant, appropriate, acceptable concepts

When developing and implementing survey instruments, researchers need to recognize that some survey items will never be "culturally sensitive." For example, while developing a list of survey items to be included in all four of the National Cancer Institute Native American cervical cancer research interventions, items asking about the last Pap smear and pelvic exam were reviewed via focus groups, Native advisory groups, and individual face-to-face interviews within American Indian, Alaska Native, and Native Hawaiian communities. After multiple revisions (approximately thirteen), the conclusion was proposed by the Native Hawaiian staff that certain survey items would never really be "culturally sensitive," because they violated the cultural norms of modesty. However, when the survey interview *protocol* was modified (to have a gentle and well trained interviewer administer the survey in a quiet, personal manner), those same items became "acceptable" to the participants, and the interviewers were able to collect accurate information. Thus, "culturally acceptable" means that the project will not be offensive to the participant and result in increased withdrawals from the study.

OBJECTIVE 2: DESCRIBE CULTURALLY COMPETENT INTERVENTIONS TO ADDRESS BARRIERS TO PARTICIPATING IN CANCER PROGRAMS

Barriers are identified in other chapters of this text. There are basically four "categories" of barriers: policy, poverty, psychosocial, and sociocultural. This next section describes some strategies for addressing the latter three categories of barriers.

INTERVENTIONS TO ADDRESS POVERTY-RELATED BARRIERS

Transportation

When developing interventions to address "poverty-related" barriers, strategies can be very generic and still have effect. Obviously, a cancer intervention cannot appropriately address the most significant poverty-related barriers (e.g., homelessness, life and health priorities other than cancer). However, it is quite feasible to provide bus tokens, taxi vouchers, or free elder van transportation for potential study participants.

Child Care

A service setting can develop a partnership with another local child care agency by which clients can leave their grandchildren or children during occasional appointments, meetings, or health procedures. Due to numerous liability issues, it is becoming less and less possible for cancer interventions to provide child care services themselves. There are strict protocols regarding criminal backgrounds of potential child care providers (i.e., requiring fingerprint verification that there have been no previous child molestation convictions), child care staff training (e.g., first aid, CPR), safety equipment, insurance coverage, kidnaping-prevention, and so on.

Unless the organization providing the cancer intervention is also licensed as a child care facility, community partnerships are a more feasible way to address these barriers to study participation.

Lack of Telephone

Telephone surveys are among the least expensive data-collection methods. However, if the community has difficulty accessing telephones, the data are of questionable value. For collecting data that is not too personal, such as on tobacco use, self-administered inventories written at an easy-to-understand literacy level have yielded valid information (Hodge et al. 1996). However, when personal data (i.e., cultural beliefs, personal medical history) are being collected, face-to-face surveys have rendered the most accurate data.

Lack of Access to Care

Lack of medical insurance or access to an Indian Health Service (IHS) facility, lack of Indian-owned and operated health program (93-638 facility), or lack of access to "compacting" services is another poverty-related barrier. When developing an intervention, alternatives need to be addressed. Many poor people are available for "indigent-care" programs if they live within designated areas. Others are available for Medicare or Medicaid. However, while conducting community-based interventions it is not unusual to lose three to six months waiting for potential Indian clients to be declared "eligible" for Medicare or Medicaid. The reason for the delay is that government agencies determine who is the "last payor," and both Medicare and IHS have this status. While implementing the NAWWA breast health project, the Native Sisters and project coordinators had to help the agencies understand that urban Indian women in our sites do not have access to, or are ineligible for, an IHS facility and therefore must be served through Medicare or Medicaid. Some social service personnel suggested that the women return to the reservation for follow-up diagnostic tests or treatment, being totally unaware of the limited availability of mammography equipment throughout IHS (14 machines nationwide), tribal nations requirements to be a current resident (to have lived on the reservation for at least six months) to be eligible for services, and the distances people who have to travel to IHS facilities. In Denver, Indian women would have to travel 350 miles to Ignacio, in the southwest corner of the state, for IHS services —and Ignacio does not provide cancer diagnostic or treatment services anyway.

This limited accessibility to services is a concern also since federal agencies, such as the National Cancer Institute, do not pay for services. The researcher has to find some way to provide access, perhaps partnerships with other organizations, or in-kind funding from a foundation that can pay for services (like the Susan G. Komen Breast Cancer Foundation, or the Breast Cancer Fund). The availability of such foundations is limited in general; those that exist may be limited to a particular cancer site. For example, there are few foundations to support colorectal screening service costs. The same is true for prostate, gallbladder, and stomach screening services.

INTERVENTIONS TO ADDRESS PSYCHO-SOCIAL BARRIERS

Making Information Easier to Understand

Communication barriers are included in this category. The most profound communication barrier is cancer information that is not understandable to the client. Many materials are developed for grade fourteen reading level but the general population functions at grade five to seven; therefore word choice and sentence structure in the informational materials must be modified. An example of making word choice more understandable is to change "participate" to "take part" and "Pap smear" to "Pap test". Such modifications are also needed in the informed-consent process, to help the participant understand what the study entails and allow for an informed decision regarding participation. Many publications are available with formulas for determining the reading level of documents, mostly counting syllables and words in sentences.

An excellent series of booklets has been released by the National Susan G. Komen Breast Cancer Foundation on developing effective cancer-education print materials for selected populations. For example, there are separate booklets for Native Americans, African Americans, Hispanics, Asian-Pacific Islanders, and lesbians. These booklets have been developed to provide culturally specific guidelines relevant to target populations (The Susan G. Komen Breast Cancer Foundation 1997).

Another example of a successful, culturally competent strategy is modification of the NCI booklets on recruitment into clinical trials. The Eastern Cooperative Oncology Group (ECOG) contracted with the AMC Cancer Research Center to make the information easy to understand and to focus-group-test various graphic layouts to determine acceptability among African-American communities. The materials were well received by African-American cancer patients. In addition, these products have been reviewed by American Indians and found to be acceptable among them as well. ECOG has been seeking funds to reproduce and disseminate these easy-to-understand informational recruitment materials.

Back-Translation

Other cancer interventions have prepared easy-to-understand messages and then translated them into another language. However, when such messages are translated—for example into Spanish—it is imperative that they be "back-translated" into English. In this way, slight variations of word choice are frequently identified. Likewise, there are multiple forms of Spanish, and the translation must be made by someone in the target community so that the appropriate form is used. For example, a cancer project in Texas in the early 1990s had the information translated into Spanish by a staff member who was fluent in Castellan Spanish;

when the back-translation process was conducted by local residents, the connotations of local Spanish as compared to Castellan Spanish were so different that the translated copy made no sense at all. A similar translation difficulty occurred on a smaller scale when materials were translated into Lakota, but the local Sioux dialect was Dakota. The resulting educational materials were unusable in the Dakota-speaking community. This illustrates the problem of "translating" ideas as well as words. Many individuals may be able to translate words but not the meanings and the related ideas.

In addition to back-translation, cancer prevention and control interventions often require the use of a translator. Within each local community the researcher needs to determine what translator programs exist. For example, some hospitals are mandated to have monies available to hire sign-language or Spanish-speaking interpreters for their patients. Such interpreters may be available for other languages (e.g., Thai, Vietnamese, and Lakota at Sioux Sans Hospital) within the target population and community.

Health System Navigators

Among the psychosocial barriers to participating in cancer prevention and control studies is fear and discomfort with Western medical facilities, such as hospitals. It is important to have some type of relaxed human contact available to an individual who has received an abnormal cancer test result. The "navigator" model evolved from an innovative patient support program implemented by Dr. Harold Freeman in Harlem Hospital (Freeman et al. 1995). The navigator is trained to accompany the patient to follow-up appointments, providing emotional support and advocacy. Navigator support is typically initiated as soon as the patient receives an abnormal cancer test result. The navigator supports and assists patients in accessing services and obtaining appropriate follow-up. Navigators have helped achieve patient compliance with recommended medical treatment as well as in increasing access to state-of-the-art treatment, for instance, to control subsequent cancers. They accompany the patient from office to office within the hospital or clinic, help complete the paperwork, and help make certain the patient understands what is happening (see Green and Werner, this volume; Burhansstipanov et al. 1998a).

INTERVENTIONS TO ADDRESS SOCIO-CULTURAL RELATED BARRIERS

Culturally Relevant Resource Materials

Many sociocultural barriers are on the subconscious level or require additional efforts to learn what they are and how they affect participation in a cancer intervention. One that is very broad-based is limited access to cancer information that is culturally relevant to the intended local population. This lack of relevance results in communities erroneously feeling that they are not susceptible to cancer or that their risk is low or nonexistent. For example, we conducted focus groups reviewing cultural educational materials with American Indians. Cancer education materials (not culture specific) were laid out on a table; we observed which materials women picked up, reviewed (i.e., appeared to read, or looked at the pictures and graphs), returned to the table, slipped into their purses, etc. We interviewed the women about cancer after they had had an opportunity to read through educational pamphlets. When queried whether cancer was a problem among Native Americans, the typical response was, "No, there was nothing in there about Indian people!" As culturally relevant educational materials were developed for specific cancer sites (e.g., cervix and breast), the women had totally different responses. We also found that materials small enough to fit within a purse were desired. Likewise, those with color and Indian graphics were much more likely to be read. Including quotes from other native women also had great effect.

Samples of educational materials that have been successfully used within native communities have been summarized in publications (Burhansstipanov and Barry 1994; Burhansstipanov and Tenney 1994); for those with access to the Internet they are listed on our Web page, http://www.aclin.org/code/nac. Of primary importance is the American Indian/Alaska Native Cancer Information Resource Center and Learning Exchange, which is accessible from Mayo Clinic (see Kaur in this volume). This resource center includes culturally relevant educational materials that have been successfully used within American Indian and Alaska Native communities throughout the United States.

Culturally Relevant Cancer Education Programs

Many of the sociocultural barriers to cancer interventions can be addressed through the development and implementation of culturally relevant educational programs. Every culture holds certain myths about cancer, and they need to be addressed in a manner that is both comfortable for and relevant to the community. Many of these can be generic educational efforts. Others cannot, and these therefore require culturally specific interventions. For example, several years ago, on the first day of mammography screening in a Southwestern Indian community, a woman was diagnosed with cancer. The community reaction was that she had been healthy when she went into the van—the machine had "given" her cancer. Local educators attempted to address this belief construct but were unsuccessful. Finally, they turned to respected Native American leaders in the community for suggestions. The conflict was resolved by having an acknowledged traditional Indian healer perform a cleansing ceremony and blessing of the machine. Women were then comfortable about participating in screening again.

Survivors as Community Lay Educators

Cancer survivors can be incredibly effective educators within the community, particularly within their own cultural groups. Successful interventions have given cancer survivors access to scientific information about cancer diagnosis, treatment, and recovery in addition to their own experiences. The visibility of these people within the community dispels many myths, of which the greatest is that a cancer diagnosis is a death sentence. Healthy survivors actively involved in community-based cancer interventions can address the misinformation. They can explain that most cancers are not familial; that a mammogram can accurately identify most tumors in older women; having a mammogram or other uncomfortable screening tests lasts only for a short while and cannot be compared with the pain of having the test too late, after cancer has spread. Survivors have extraordinary credibility and acceptability within the community. Trained survivors have been included in many successful interventions, including "Sister-to-Sister" and "Á Su Salud." The survivors are invaluable in helping others who are newly diagnosed *and their families* understand the diagnosis and treatment protocols.

Many survivors from medically underserved communities, like Native Americans, continue to live in poverty. It is very appropriate to pay cancer survivors during their training and while working on cancer prevention and control interventions. The previous norm was simply to have people volunteer their time, but the survivor still has a family to feed and probably also needs paid employment. Survivors who live in poverty and are not paid frequently do their best to work with the cancer program, but turnover is very high, because they eventually have to have a paying job. A very valuable staff member is lost, and the effort of training her is wasted.

Training Providers

This and related barriers have been targeted by the Network for Cancer Prevention and Control Research among American Indian and Alaska Native Populations (see Kaur, this volume) in both the federal and state strategic plans (Hampton 1996). Recommended actions include educating providers on the growing prevalence of cancer among American Indians and Alaska Natives. When feasible, it is helpful to offer continuing medical education units for such training. The cancer prevention and control study needs to provide resources or training to help providers understand cultural issues that influence participation in local interventions. Such training may include having the provider practice explaining complex procedures so that they are understandable to the patient. The tests, examinations, and protocols need to be explained in a way that addressess patients' fear, by helping them understand what is being done to them.

Need for Accurate Data to Educate Both Providers and Community

As has been published in the Network for Cancer Prevention and Control Research among American Indian and·Alaska Native Populations' national and state strategic plans, there is a research priority for collecting and reporting racially specific data. This recommendation has been included in other publications (Hampton 1989, 1992; Burhansstipanov 1994, 1995, 1996; Burhans-stipanov and Dresser 1993; Burhansstipanov and Tenney 1995; Burhansstipanov et al. 1998b).

As a result of data errors, providers are misinformed about the significance of cancer within specific native communities (e.g., Northern Plains) and are less aggressive in their efforts to identify and refer cancer symptoms. Federal agencies, such as the National Cancer Institute (NCI), *until recent years* was likely to discount cancer as a problem, because the primary sources for their data summaries are from Arizona and New Mexico—where Native American cancer incidence and mortality rates are lower than for Indian communities in other parts of the United States (Burhansstipanov 1997). The optimal strategy for addressing these issues is to collect local cancer data to help the community and provider understand the types of cancer that are of most relevance in their setting.

Cultural Belief Structures

Local cultural nuances are not taught in books; the researcher, health educator, or provider must work directly with the community so that *local* beliefs, rather than beliefs of a tribe living in another region, are the focus (see Weiner, this volume). For example, "discussing cancer" is regarded as a form of *spreading* the disease among some Southwestern tribes, but less so among Northern Plains tribes. If the cancer study is being conducted in the Northern Plains, it is culturally inappropriate to stress educational interventions about spreading the cancer spirit. Some beliefs are very challenging to address in a culturally competent manner and can best be addressed with local leadership and guidance. For example, the belief that the Creator is punishing the cancer patient for some wrong performed in the past is very delicate. Different tribes address this quite differently. In one instance, a family in a Southwestern tribe worked with a traditional Indian healer in a cleansing and healing ceremony for the entire family (since all members were affected by the cancer and were thought to be partially responsible for the cancer growth). In another community, the patient was an active member of the Native American Church, and the people who took part in the religious ceremony all prayed for guidance from the Creator for his recovery. Others, such as Mary P. Lovato, experienced a vision of the work she was supposed to do (see Kaur in this volume for a description of Mary's "Gathering of Cancer Support" training program). Through her training programs, participants learn that cancer has no prejudices and afflicts people of all walks of life, good and bad alike.

Ceremonies

A few well-intentioned researchers, public health educators, and service providers have attempted to combine traditional Indian ceremonies with cancer prevention and control programs. Basically, ceremonies are private and need to be respected for their spiritualism. The preparation needed to conduct a ceremony "in the good way" needs to remain private and under the traditional Indian healers' control. Cancer interventions that adapt such ceremonies *may be* regarded as "bastardizing" a religious ceremony and be avoided (Burhansstipanov 1998). Researchers who wish to collaborate with traditional Indian healers need to ensure that the healer's words and guidance are followed. When a ceremony is to be modified, to include educational sessions or in some other purpose, the name of the event needs to be changed so that local members of the community realize it. For example, during the NAWWA Traditional Support Circles in Denver, the Native Sisters would have topics for each circle, such as self-esteem. They would introduce the topic and do some self-esteem exercises together; then each of the women would talk about their self-identity before and after the cancer diagnosis. Much of the latter format was similar to that of a "Talking Circle," but some of the initial activities were too different to be a true "Talking Circle." For example, one is prohibited from discussing anything learned in a "Talking Circle" outside of that gathering, whereas the Native Sisters wanted the women to feel free to share what they had learned with others. Women may be asked to go home and talk with their families about how the family members felt about the woman before and after being diagnosed with breast cancer; how the woman's breast cancer diagnosis affected family members' own self-esteem—husbands and children feeling helpless, powerless, and as having lowered self-esteem. By calling it a "Traditional Support Circle," they were not violating total privacy mandates associated with the "Talking Circle." Women still were prohibited from sharing any other woman's story discussed during the Circle unless she gave permission to do so.

Addressing the Need for Native Providers and Researchers

These sociocultural barriers may be addressed through a variety of mechanisms, some of which require years to mature. Much of the fear of white doctors is due to the dearth of physicians of color. There needs to be a way to bring in young American Indian premed and medical students as investigators or assistants to investigators on research projects, so that Indian providers learn about cancer prevention and control research. This approach helps to train the next generation of cancer researchers and increases the likelihood that those providers will have a greater depth of understanding of the local American Indian cultures. To have access to Western medical care that offers providers of many colors, rather than primarily white, will help dispel the myths of cancer spread by whites.

Modesty

Modesty issues affect both American Indian women *and* men. Interventions may include such provider protocols as asking the patient how to make her or him more comfortable. One Indian woman wanted a separate bed sheet to cover her face; she did not want to see the provider. Many women and men have a preference regarding the sex of their provider; women usually prefer a woman provider for the Pap test. Obviously, a cancer prevention and control study that can offer providers of both sexes is of great assistance in allowing the patient to choose his or her provider. This helps to address modesty issues, but few programs have sufficient monies to do this. Another way to address modesty issues has been initiated by Mary Alice Trapp, RN, who trains nurses on women's health examinations. Her technique is to ask the woman if she would prefer to remain partially clothed during her pelvic examination (i.e., leave on her bra and blouse). During the clinical breast examination, the patient is allowed the option of putting on her skirt or slacks to cover her lower body (personal communication, Trapp 1997).

As another example, we had a woman client who wanted to have her husband with her, standing by her head while the cancer screening and diagnostic tests were being conducted. During focus groups with Indian men during 1997, the men were adamant that they not be embarrassed during cancer screening tests, especially digital examinations. Some felt that the tests would have been less violating had the provider explained what he was doing, so that the men understood that he was not doing anything unethical. Other men said that they would prefer to have a female provider do the digital exam; they were more concerned about "homophobia" issues than with modesty, and the woman had the additional benefit of having smaller hands than a male.

Combination of Western Medicine with Traditional Indian Healing

The combination of two healing systems can be an incredibly successful intervention. Some providers have implemented these types of teams for several years; their cancer patients appear to have less anxiety and greater spiritual strength to undergo the rigor of chemotherapy or radiation. The Indian cancer patients who participate in some form of spiritual healing have more positive outlooks on their lives after cancer treatment. Some interventions require negotiation with the hospital. For example, a Northwestern cancer patient wanted a particular ceremony performed prior to surgery; this was to be conducted in his room and to involve the burning of sage, cedar, and other similar items. The hospital had a strict no-smoking policy and felt that this burning of plant products violated the state ordinance. The research team had to work with the hospital staff and legal advisors. To protect other patients from the "potentially harmful burned product," the doors to the patient's room were sealed and the windows opened. The hospital ventilation to that room was temporarily shut off. Other patients were notified of what was to occur in case they smelled anything unusual.

Traditional Indian healing appears to be a successful complementary therapy to Western medical technology and to provide excellent spiritual healing and recovery for both the patient and the entire family. In contrast, Weiner's study among southern California tribal communities showed that some individuals who only used biomedicine were also positive about treatments and outcomes (Weiner 1997).

OBJECTIVE 3: DESCRIBE AT LEAST TWO SUCCESSFULLY CULTURALLY COMPETENT COMMUNITY INTERVENTIONS FOR CANCER PREVENTION AND CONTROL

Cancer interventions are described in a variety of publications. The October 1996 Supplement issue of *Cancer* highlights several culturally competent Native American cancer interventions. The October/November/December 1993 issue of *Alaska Medicine* includes descriptions of interventions highlighted during the "Cancer in Indian Country" National Native American Cancer conference. *American Indian Culture and Research Journal* (volume 16, number 3, 1992) highlights papers and interventions described during the 1989 First National Conference on Cancer in Native Americans. Native American cancer interventions are also briefly described in this volume in Dr. Judith Kaur's chapter, as well as in Cunningham-Sabo's and Davis' chapter.

This section includes a few other projects that have not yet been highlighted in those other chapters or publications.

Native Sisters

The Native Women's Wellness through Awareness (NAWWA) project staff modified the Health Systems Navigators' role to be culturally relevant to American Indians (Burhansstipanov et al. 1998a). The navigators of the NAWWA were called "Native Sisters." Native Sisters are American Indian women trained to provide emotional support to American Indian women throughout the screening and follow-up procedures. *The greatest difference* between the Native Sisters and other Navigator programs is that the latter start work when the patient receives an abnormal cancer test. In contrast, Native Sisters focus their attention on recruitment for screening. Obviously, if women were not being screened, they would never have the opportunity to have their cancers diagnosed early for Native Sisters to provide support. Unlike most other navigator programs, the Native Sisters gradually became more and more involved in the initial recruitment to screening itself as well as in a leadership role for all subsequent project components (see Figure 13.1).

NAWWA Native Sisters' Roles

The NAWWA implemented a broad variety of recruitment strategies, but clearly the personal approach of the Native Sisters was regarded as the most effective by clients (as assessed by postscreening self-administered inventory). The Sisters take leadership roles in recruiting women for screening and are present on the day of screening, to attempt to make the experience less traumatic for the American Indian patient. Among the advantages of having the Native Sisters involved in the initial screening was that because the clients had an opportunity to become acquainted with them when no trauma (abnormal breast test) was present, a sense of comfort and trust developed. This made follow-up contact more comfortable and less stressful than it would have been if the initial contact with the Native Sisters had occurred after receiving abnormal test results. A detailed description of the Native Sisters has been published clarifying some of the responsibilities (Burhansstipanov et al. 1998a). Of greatest importance is the adaptability of the Native Sisters to different tribes, as well as to other underserved populations.

Native American Cancer Researchers Training Program

The Native American Cancer Researchers Training differs significantly from previously described cancer interventions, in that it is designed to have outcomes several years in the future. This is a National Cancer Institute investigator-initiated award, designed to identify and train the next generation of Native American cancer researchers. Through this project, Native Americans are recruited who are interested in learning more about research or learning more about *cancer* research (i.e., switching their current research emphasis from alcohol or diabetes to cancer). Candidates submit brief applications, as well as letters of support from their employers, who must agree to allow up to four weeks' absence from work to participate in the training. The project requires two to three weeks intensive training during early summer, followed by one week of intensive follow-up training during the fall. Through innovative support of NCI staff during summer 1997, funding was made available in small amounts for research trainees to conduct pilot tests. This allocation to young researchers has been received with great enthusiasm, and such encouragement increases the likelihood of remaining in the field of cancer research. The preliminary outcomes from this training intervention is very positive; the actual effectiveness will be evident many years from now, when the participants are recipients of investigator-initiated research grants from the NCI.

OBJECTIVE 4: BRIEFLY DESCRIBE GENERALIZABILITY ISSUES OF "SUCCESSFUL" INTERVENTIONS

Researchers and service providers eagerly attempt to duplicate successful cancer prevention and control interventions in their local area, and they are sometimes surprised by the results. An intervention can be very effective in one subpopulation, in one geographic setting, but ineffective in the "same" subpopulation in another geographic setting. For instance, African-American church leadership in a cancer intervention can "work" in Atlanta and be ineffective in the African-American churches of New York. There are multiple explanations for the variable effect, or translatableness, of successful interventions, but the most obvious is that local communities have characteristics unique to their own setting and that those characteristics must be addressed when replicating an intervention.

Cultural Modification of "Replicable Successful Interventions"

When working with medically underserved populations, most researchers and service providers find that a "replicable successful intervention" requires local community leadership to modify the intervention so as to be culturally competent in their local area. Although this process is met with skepticism by behavioral-medicine scientists, it is the difference of working in a lab and working with real people in community settings. While modifying, it is important to keep as much of the original protocol in place, so that it is possible to compare results. For example, in the National Heart Lung and Blood Institute Pathways project, designed to reduce obesity in American Indian children, one segment of the protocol included traditional storytelling. The model story was about "Coyote" and his trickster behaviors; it required a young person to decide between sharing food and gluttony. The original story is from the Southwest, and it would have little impact delivered to an Indian child living on the East Coast or the Northwest. Both areas have similar stories, with the same theme, but with characters common in their region; the fox is the trickster on the East Coast, and the raven in the Northwest. To be culturally relevant, the stories needed to be relevant to the geographic region of the country. Rather than being strict with the protocol and demanding that exactly the same story (which would not have had the desired outcome) be used in all geographic settings, the protocol was allowed to keep the same concepts but be culturally relevant (for additional information, see Davis and Cunningham-Sabo, in this volume).

Collaborative Partnerships with other Organizations May Be Unattainable

Sometimes interventions are not replicable because there are conditions inherent in one region that cannot effectively be duplicated in another. Among the more successful cancer interventions is in a specific Southwestern tribe, in New Mexico. The intervention has been very effective in screening women for breast cancer. However, when other communities *outside* of New Mexico have attempted to replicate the project, they have been unable to do so. This is due to the model tribe's having a very productive, conducive working partnership between the Indian Health Service, the New Mexico Tumor Registry (and the New Mexico Comprehensive Cancer Center), and the Cancer Prevention and Control Program of New Mexico. This partnership has resulted in collaborative efforts to recruit and screen women in culturally comfortable settings; it is an excellent program. People attempting to replicate this program in a state other than New Mexico, however, found that there were limited or no IHS services available, no comprehensive cancer center or tumor registry in partnership, and no support for screening from the state cancer prevention and control program. The model New Mexico Indian project has successfully been replicated in other communities *within* New Mexico, which has the highest compliance with breast and cervical cancer screening among Native Americans of any state (CDC 1997).

Similar Approaches May Be Met with Resistance by Intended Collaborators

An intervention can be very effective in one underserved population but ineffective in another. For example, Sister-to-Sister has been very well received among many African-American communities, and it relies on close collaboration with local churches. When attempting to replicate this program with Native American churches, there was great annoyance at the attempt to tie cancer to spiritual ceremonies.

Population Density or Isolation May Affect the Replication Model

Á Su Salud is another incredibly successful intervention within Hispanic and Latina populations. This intervention relies on local communities leaders to initiate one-on-one cancer education with their neighbors. Cancer survivors canvass the neighborhoods to educate others about the benefits of early detection. However, Indian populations tend to be scattered throughout the urban area (rarely do one or two census tracks isolate the majority of the urban Indian population) or to live in isolated areas in rural communities or reservations. Distance and availability of survivors or advocates to implement Á Su Salud face to face mean that the program has more effect in New Mexico and Arizona, where American Indian communities are easier to identify, than in other regions and reservations around the country.

CONCLUSION

Researchers and service providers need to proceed with cancer prevention, control interventions, and replication models with patience and respect for medically underserved populations. This chapter primarily focuses on Native Americans, but most communities can identify culturally relevant examples for their local setting. Underserved and underscreened populations, such as Native Americans, think differently about health and health care. This is not "ignorance" but rather life perceptions and life priorities that differ from the Western medical model. These differences *should* be addressed prior to introduction of an intervention being introduced in a medically underserved community (Orthodox Jewish women, Native Americans, poor whites, African Americans, Latinos and Hispanics, Cambodians, Thais, etc.). Community-based interventions require more time than many other types of interventions, but they tend to remain in the community long after funding ceases to be available, to result in the training of local people with new skills that can be used for other projects, to be innovative, creative and dynamic. It is rewarding and beneficial work.

LITERATURE CITED

Burhansstipanov L. 1995. Native American Data Limitations and Home Care. *Alaska Medicine* 37(4):133–138.

—. 1997. *Cancer Among Elder Native Americans*. Native Elder Health Care Resource Center, University of Colorado Health Sciences Center, Denver, CO.

—. 1998. Native American cancer programs: Recommendations for increased support. *Cancer Supplement* 83 (October 15) (8).

Burhansstipanov, L., D. Bad Wound, N. Capelouto, F. Goldfarb, L. Harjo, L. Hatathlie, G. Vigil, and M. White. 1998a. Native Sister, Culturally Relevant "Navigator" Patient-Support. *Cancer Practice* 6(3): 191–194.

Burhansstipanov, L., and K. C. Barry. 1994. *Cancer education resources for American Indians and Alaska Natives.* NIH Pub. No. 94–3706. Bethesda, MD: National Cancer Institute.

Burhansstipanov L., M. B. Dignan, D. Bad Wound, N. Capelouto, F. Goldfarb, L. Harjo, L. Hatathalie, M. Tenney, G. Vigil, and M. White. 1998b. Native American recruitment into breast cancer screening: The NAWWA Project. Submiited to *Journal of Cancer Education.*

Burhansstipanov, L., and Dresser, C. M. 1993. *Native American Monograph #1: Documentation of the cancer research needs of American Indians and Alaska Natives.* NIH Pub. No. 93-3603. Bethesda, MD: National Cancer Institute.

Burhansstipanov, L., and S. Morris. 1998. Breast cancer screening among American Indians and Alaska Natives. *Federal Practitioner: For the Health Care Professions of the VA, DOD, and PHS* 15(1):12–25.

Burhansstipanov, L., and M. Tenney. 1994. American Indian/Alaska Native Cancer Resources. *Cancer Practices* 2(6):447–449.

—. 1995. Native American Public Health issues. *Current Issues in Public Health* 1(1):35–41.

Centers for Disease Control. 1997. *Reaching women for mammography screening: Successful strategies of the Naional Breast and Cervical Cancer Early Detection Program,* August.

Freeman, H. P., B. J. Muth, and J. F. Kerner. 1995. Expanding access to cancer screening and clinical follow-up among the medically underserved. *Cancer Practice* (January–February) 3(1):19–30.

Hampton, J. W. 1989. The heterogeneity of cancer in Native American populations. In *Minorities and Cancer,* ed. L. A. Jones, 45–53. New York: Springer–Verlag.

—. 1992. Cancer prevention and control in American Indians and Alaska Natives. *American Indian Culture and Research Journal* 16:41–49.

—. 1996. Overview of National Cancer Institute networks for cancer control research in Native American populations. *Cancer Supplement* 78(7):1545–1552.

Hodge, F. S., L. Fredericks, and P. Kipnis. 1996. Patient and smoking patterns in northern California American Indian clinics: Urban and rural contracts. *Cancer Supplement* 78(7):1623–1628.

The Susan G. Komen Breast Cancer Foundation. 1997. *Native Americans: Developing effective cancer education print materials.* Dallas: The Susan G. Komen Breast Cancer Foundation.

Weiner, D. 1997. Personal Communication.

Figure 13.1
NAWWA Native Sisters' Roles

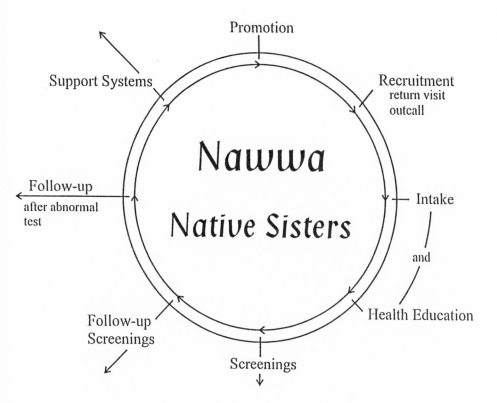

Chapter 14

Physical Activity and Cancer in Hispanic Populations: Is There a Relationship?

Lisa K. Staten

Cancer is one of the leading causes of death for Hispanic[1] populations in the United States, second only to heart disease (Ramirez et al. 1995). Despite this fact, information pertaining to cancer incidence rates and risk factors in U.S. Hispanics is extremely rare (Trapido et al. 1995). Although Hispanic men and women experience types of cancer similar to those of non-Hispanic whites, site-specific incidence rates tend to be lower (American Cancer Society 1997). Regional differences in incidence rates emphasize the heterogeneity of the Hispanic population (Trapido et al. 1995). Therefore, the differences between U.S. Hispanics and non-Hispanic whites in incidence rates cannot be explained solely by genetics.

Environmental and behavioral factors are extremely important contributors to cancer risk. The importance of lifestyle factors is reflected in the mortality rate for colon and rectum cancers in males in the United States (all ethnic groups combined) compared to Mexico; cancer statistics between 1988 and 1991 show the rate was more than five times higher in the United States. The rate for U.S. females was approximately four times higher than for Mexican females. Per 100,000 people, there were 16.7 male deaths and 11.4 female deaths in the United States, compared to 3.3 male deaths and 3.1 female deaths in Mexico (American Cancer Society 1994). Groups of new immigrants from Mexico exhibit the Mexican rate, but the rate of colon cancer in Mexican Americans living in the United States appears to be increasing (Savitz 1986) and may eventually mirror the rates of the non-Hispanic white population. In attempts to understand why these differences occur, various patterns of behavior have come under scrutiny. Behavioral patterns such as diet, smoking, sexual history, and more recently physical activity, have been targeted. However, the connection between physical activity and cancer risk in Hispanic populations has not received much attention. In non-Hispanic white populations, links have been argued between colon and breast cancer and physical activity levels (Bernstein et al. 1994; Martinez et al. 1997).

Hispanic women, like Asian and Native American women, are an extremely important group to study if we are to understand whether there is a link between physical activity, one and breast cancer. Although Hispanic women have lower incidence rates of breast cancer, their mortality rates from breast cancer are high compared to those of other ethnic groups with similar incidence rates (Miller et al. 1996).

This chapter will focus on issues relating to physical activity and cancer in U.S. Hispanic populations. First the chapter provides a definition of the term "physical activity" that emphasizes the relationship between physical activity and cancer. Second, the chapter examines methods for assessing physical activity and how Hispanic populations have been included. Third and most significantly, the chapter discusses issues relevant to culturally competent assessment of physical activity in Hispanic populations.

DEFINITION OF PHYSICAL ACTIVITY

The U.S. Surgeon General's recent report on physical activity (U.S. Department of Health and Human Services 1996) has increased awareness of the relationship between physical activity and health, and it highlights an explosion of programs aimed at increasing the activity levels of the United States population— for example, the PACE and CATCH projects. Project PACE (Physician-Based Assessment and Counseling for Exercise) is a San Diego County, California, program aimed at training ethnically diverse physicians to provide physical-activity counseling to their patients (Calfas et al. 1996). The CATCH program (Child and Adolescent Trial for Cardiovascular Health) targets third to fifth-grade children from ninety-six schools in four states: (Texas, Minnesota, Louisiana, and California), including children from a variety of ethnic groups (Perry et al. 1990). This school-based project incorporated programs (1991–1994) in healthy eating, physical activity, and nonsmoking in order to reduce such cardiovascular risk factors as serum lipids and lipoproteins, high blood pressure, and poor physical fitness. The program also included a family component, which promoted adult participation. The level of adult participation had a significant impact on minority students' knowledge and beliefs about physical activity, but not on their behavior. Additionally the knowledge and beliefs of boys were more affected than girls' by parental participation (Nader et al. 1996).

Physical activity is defined in the Surgeon General's report (U.S. Department of Health and Human Services 1996) as any movement produced by the contraction of skeletal muscle that increases energy expenditure above that required by the body at rest. This includes all activities beyond resting—such as household chores, leisure time activities, and work-related behaviors.

The term "physical activity" is very confusing to many. In my research into the development of culturally appropriate physical activity questionnaires, I have conducted focus groups with female Mexican-American community health workers in Nogales, Arizona, and participants of the Women's Health Initiative in Tucson, Arizona, concerning physical activity. Discussions regarding what the term means focused on aerobics and jogging, indicating that the term is strongly linked in the women's minds to activities that expend high levels of energy. Anecdotal data indicates that this interpretation is also common in non-Hispanic white populations. This misinterpretation may lead to difficulties in promoting and recruiting participants into a physical activity intervention program. Using the term as it is defined above allows researchers to examine all levels of physical activity. In fact, there is strong evidence, which will be discussed later in this paper, that links low levels of physical activity to increased risk for colon cancer. If research projects focused only on extremely high energy-expenditure activities, this association might be missed.

There are numerous methods to assess physical activity: doubly labeled water, indirect calorimetry, direct calorimetry, heart-rate monitoring, motion sensors, activity records, and activity recalls (or questionnaires). These methods can be divided into technological measures of activity, activity records (diaries), and recalls (questionnaires).

The technological measures include: doubly labeled water, indirect and direct calorimetry, heart rate monitoring, and motion sensors. Doubly labeled water is the current "gold standard" for measuring activity in terms of energy expenditure. A participant is given a "cocktail" of nonradioactive stable isotopes of hydrogen (deuterium) and oxygen (^{18}O). In adults, urine is collected prior to the cocktail, again first thing in the morning the day after the cocktail, then again at various time points throughout the following one-to-two-week period. The concentration of isotopes in the urine is used to calculate the total energy for that period (Montoye et al. 1996). With this method, differences between dietary intake and energy expenditure can be examined to assess activity levels of participants. Unfortunately, the method is relatively intrusive, extremely expensive, and not suitable for large-scale studies or intervention programs.

Direct calorimetry involves placing an individual in a specially designed metabolic chamber, where heat production, oxygen consumption, and carbon dioxide production are measured. From these measurements, absolute energy expenditure can be determined for the individual during his or her stay in the metabolic chamber (Brooks and Fahey 1985). This method is extremely expensive, the facilities are rare, and the confinement drastically interferes with an individual's normal, daily behaviors. A third method, indirect calorimetry, consists of wearing a bulky apparatus which can calculate actual energy expenditure in specific activities. The apparatus includes a mouthpiece, nose clip, Douglas Bag (a large balloonlike bag), and equipment for analyzing respired air (Montoye et al. 1996). This method is not very useful for determining a daily pattern, as it is bulky and can be uncomfortable. It is more intrusive than doubly labeled water, which only requires a drink and collection of urine.

A fourth method is heart-rate monitoring, wherein an individual wears an elastic chest strap with a receiver attached, and a heart watch. The heart rate can be recorded and then reviewed for distinct periods at various levels of activity to see when and how often people are active (U.S. Department of Health and Human Services 1996). There are several problems with this method. Emotional state affects heart rate, electrical interference and other heart watches can distort reception, and the relationship between heart rate and energy expenditure is not very good for sedentary activities.The final technological measure is the motion sensor. Motion sensors are small pieces of equipment, attached to participants' belts or worn in waist pouches, that detect motion in multiple directions. These instruments are used to look at movement patterns. Prices range from under twenty-five dollars to $500.

The technological measures tend to be expensive, invasive in varying degrees, and to interfere in normal daily activities. Nevertheless, nutritionists, exercise physiologists, and anthropologists sometimes employ such methods when looking at energy balance in individuals and populations; they are perceived as the most precise techniques, as they do not rely on participant recall or recording abilities.

Activity records require literate and extremely cooperative participants. The participants are generally asked to keep a log of their activities over a given period, ranging from one day to a week. These records are extremely time-intensive and can interfere with participant activities. Activity recalls are the tools most commonly used by epidemiologists and in clinical trials. Recalls generally consist of questions regarding specific types of activities. Questionnaire length can range from one question to hour-long interviews. The time frame ranges from one day to a lifetime. Activity recalls are relatively inexpensive, less time-consuming to administer than logs, and tend not to effect participant activity patterns. The limitations are that most questionnaires have been developed and tested in white, generally male, middle-to-upper-class populations (Marcus et al. 1995). Very few questionnaires have actually been validated for minority populations. Importantly, most activity questionnaires have been developed to examine relationships with cardiovascular disease and diabetes (see Kriska et al. 1990; Sidney et al. 1991). Few, if any, have been designed specifically for cancer research.

Epidemiological studies have looked at physical activity in a variety of ways, including focusing on different types, frequencies, and durations of activities. The majority of questionnaires have attempted to quantify either leisure activities (such as Taylor et al. 1978; Paffenbarger et al. 1978; Godin and Shephard 1985; Salonen and Lakka 1987; Kohl et al. 1988; Jacobs et al. 1989; Kriska et al. 1990; Caspersen et al. 1991) or occupation-related activities (Montoye 1971), or sometimes both (Baecke et al. 1982; Kriska and Bennett 1992; Lakka and Salonen 1992). Fewer include household chores and gardening (Bouchard et al. 1983; DiPietro et al. 1993; Washburn et al. 1993). Most studies looking at the relationship between physical activity and disease have primarily involved middle-aged to elderly middle-to-upper-socioeconomic-level white men; a few have centered on older, middle-to-upper-socioeconomic-level white women. In many cases, it is unclear whether the relationships hold true for other white females or other ethnic groups.

CANCER AND HISPANIC POPULATIONS

The five most common cancer sites for Hispanic men and women are prostate, breast, lung, and colon and rectum—the same as for non-Hispanic whites (American Cancer Society 1997). The prevalence rate of prostate, breast, lung, and colon and rectum cancer in Hispanics is approximately 30% lower than that for whites (American Cancer Society 1997). In the case of cervical cancer, Hispanic women have the highest rate, second only to Vietnamese women (American Cancer Society 1997). When compared to Mexicans and the general U.S. population, Mexican Americans exhibit an intermediate rate for many types of cancer, higher than Mexicans but lower than the general U.S. population.

Due to the heterogeneity of the people included in the term "Hispanic", some regional differences in incidence rates do appear. In a summary of cancer registry records and research articles from regions of California, Texas, Florida, Colorado, New York, Puerto Rico, New Mexico, Illinois, and Florida, Trapido and associates (1995) discovered that for men the top two cancers, lung and prostate, were consistent cross-regionally. By region, the incidence rate for Hispanic men was always lower than that for non-Hispanic men, but when compared between regions, Hispanic men in New Mexico had higher rates of prostate cancer than non-Hispanic men in New York, Texas, or Illinois. The top five sites for cancer in women matched for Hispanic and non-Hispanic women in more regions than for men. A similar pattern was seen in that Hispanic women in Illinois had higher incidence rates than non-Hispanic women in Texas, Florida, or New Mexico. This pattern indicates a strong role for environmental and behavioral factors, in addition to possible genetic factors.

PHYSICAL ACTIVITY AND CANCER

The relationship between physical activity and cancer risk appears to vary by site. Types of cancer studied in conjunction with physical activity include breast (Zheng et al 1993; Dorgan et al. 1994; Thune et al. 1997), endometrial (Shu et al. 1993), prostate (Hsing et al. 1994), stomach (Stukonis and Doll 1969), colon (Fredriksson et al. 1989; Lee et al. 1989; Benito et al. 1990; Kune et al. 1990; Slattery et al. 1990; Kono et al. 1991; Lee et al. 1991; Thun et al. 1992; Paffenbarger et al. 1993), and cancer in general (Dosemeci et al. 1993). The two forms of cancer that have been most closely linked to levels of physical activity are colon and breast. The evidence is strong for a link between low levels of current physical activity and increased risk for colon cancer (Fredriksson et al. 1989; Lee et al. 1989; Benito et al. 1990; Kune et al. 1990; Slattery et al. 1990; Kono et al. 1991; Lee et al. 1991; Thun et al. 1992; Vetter et al. 1992; Paffenbarger et al. 1993; Vineis et al. 1993; Martinez et al. 1997). Assessment of physical activity in colon cancer has included occupational activity, current leisure activities, and activities during early adulthood. The majority of studies of current occupational activity and leisure activities found a significant relationship between sedentary activity patterns and increased risk for colon cancer. Not all studies have been able to identify this association (Vetter et al. 1992; Arbman et al. 1993; Vineis et al. 1993). None of the studies of activity during early adulthood found a significant relationship (Paffenbarger et al. 1987; Marcus et al. 1994). Very few of these studies have controlled for socioeconomic conditions or diet (U.S. Department of Health and Human Services 1996). Few, if any, studies have looked at physical activity in Hispanic populations to see if low rates of physical activity are correlated with increased colon cancer risk. Hispanic participants are included in studies but do not constitute a large percentage of the participants, due to their lower incidence rate of colon cancer.

The relationship between physical activity and breast cancer is less clear. Studies of physical activity and breast cancer have focused on many different types and timings of participation in activity, such as current occupational activities (Vena et al. 1987; Zheng et al. 1993 Thune et al. 1997), leisure activities (Bernstein et al. 1994; Dorgan et al. 1994; Thune et al. 1997), and activity levels during childhood, adolescence, and early adulthood. Results have not been consistent. To date, virtually no studies have been conducted with Hispanic women on this matter, with the exception of an epidemiological survey looking at two physical-activity questions and reports of cancer incidence (Albanes et al. 1989).

Many of the difficulties and inconsistencies involved in associations between current levels of physical activity (within the past year) may be due to the use of assessment tools that are not comparable, lack of control for socioeconomic conditions, ethnicity and other confounders, and the extreme difficulty of designing a measure of activity patterns for childhood, adolescence, and young adulthood that can be validated. The only means for validating a measurement of lifetime or past physical activity is to conduct a long-term cohort study. Data on physical activity patterns of young girls of all ethnic groups needs to be collected at regular intervals, beginning prior to puberty and following through middle age. Unfortunately, this type of study is extremely expensive and requires a series of investigators to complete.

Although the exploration of the relationship between physical activity and cancer is in its early stages, the American Cancer Society (ACS) has included increasing levels of physical activity in its recommendations to reduce cancer risk. ACS states that it is important to be physically active in order to balance caloric intake with energy expenditure, and it links physical activity to colon, rectum, prostate, endometrium, breast (postmenopausal) and kidney cancers, though it does not define what is meant by physical activity nor inactivity (American Cancer Society 1998). ACS guidelines are distributed to the general public through public service announcements and through doctors' offices, via pamphlets. Many of their brochures are available in Spanish and English.

PHYSICAL ACTIVITY IN HISPANIC POPULATIONS

In June 1997 the journal *Medicine and Science in Sports and Exercise* published a supplemental issue entitled "A Collection of Physical Activity Questionnaires for Health-Related Research" (Pereira et al. 1997). Very few validation and reliability studies of physical-activity questionnaires mention Hispanic or Latino participants (Garcia-Palmieri et al. 1982; Shea et al. 1991; Rauh et al. 1992; Sallis et al. 1993). Nonetheless, there is a great deal of data from national surveys, but the surveys have not been validated.

As indicated above, ethnic differences in activity patterns have not been considered. In fact, minority populations are rarely included in these cancer studies. In light of the lower incidence rates of many types of cancer in most minority populations, it is noteworthy that Hispanics have been documented as having lower levels of physical activity than non-Hispanic whites in all national surveys. Based on the results of three national surveys (the Behavioral Risk Factor Surveillance System [BRFSS], the National Health Interview Survey [NHIS], and the Third National Health and Nutrition Examination Survey [NHANES III]), the U.S. Surgeon General's report (U.S. Department of Health and Human Services 1996) states the following: "Physical inactivity is more prevalent among women than men, among blacks and Hispanics than whites, among older than younger adults, and among the less affluent than the more affluent (1996, 8)."

Due to the results of these surveys, the *Healthy People 2000* objectives have set different goals for Hispanic populations. One of the objectives is to increase to 30% the proportion of people aged six and older who engage regularly, preferably daily, in light to moderate physical activity for at least thirty minutes per day; for Hispanics aged eighteen and older, the goal is to increase the proportion to at least 25%. Current estimates place Hispanic populations at approximately 20%, versus non-Hispanic whites at 24%. National surveys from the early 1990s estimate that 16.5% to 18.9% of Hispanic women participate in regular, sustained physical activity five or more times per week (National Health Interview Survey 1991[NHIS] and Behavioral Risk Factor Surveillance System 1992 [BRFSS], cited in U.S. Department of Health and Human Services 1996).

A second *Healthy People 2000* objective is to reduce to no more than 15% the proportion of people aged six and older who engage in no leisure-time physical activity at all. For Hispanics the *Healthy People 2000* goal is to reduce this proportion to no more than 25%. Current estimates of the percentage of U.S. Hispanics engaging in no leisure-time physical activity range from 29.1% to 43.8; the highest rates are for Hispanic females. In all national surveys since the early 1990s, socioeconomic conditions have been a strong factor in indicating who is exercising and who is not. The lower the income level, the lower the participation in moderate physical activity (U.S. Department of Health and Human Services 1996). One of the major flaws in the national surveys is that they focus almost exclusively on leisure-time activities. In low socioeconomic-level populations, individuals may be precluded by the financial and occupational demands on their time from exercising in their leisure time, but they may be performing strenuous activities on the job. Are Hispanic populations really less active, or is it an artifact of the tools used to measure activity?

DEVELOPMENT AND SELECTION OF APPROPRIATE
ASSESSMENT TOOLS

Prior to embarking on a study examining the relationship between physical activity and cancer in Hispanic populations, more studies are needed to validate the cultural sensitivity of the instruments currently in use. The most comprehensive testing of questionnaires in an Hispanic group was by Rauh et al. (1992), who validated six questionnaires with a group of forty-five middle-class, bicultural Latinos. The authors state that the same questionnaires need to be validated in low-socioeconomic individuals who are not bicultural before many generalizations can be made for the Hispanic population as a whole. Despite this comment, the authors supported the use of standard physical activity questionnaires in Hispanic populations.

At the University of Arizona, I am in the process of validating a physical activity questionnaire, the Spanish Arizona activity frequency questionnaire (AAFQ). The AAFQ was initially designed, like many others, for a group of middle to upper-middle-class, white, non-Hispanic individuals participating in a study of colon cancer at the Arizona Cancer Center. The AAFQ includes a wide range of activities, including occupational, leisure, household, and recreational ones. In an attempt to make the instrument more culturally sensitive, I have conducted the focus groups mentioned earlier to determine which activities are superfluous and which activities should be added. No activities were deemed superfluous, and several activities including childcare and adult care were added. We have completed an initial pilot validation study comparing AAFQ results with doubly labeled water results in a sample of six middle-class Hispanic women. The next step is to do a larger-scale validation study, using a larger sample of women from varying socioeconomic statuses, including both urban and rural dwellers. Following this study, we will expand the validation studies to Hispanic males.

During the redesign and piloting of the Spanish AAFQ, several issues have arisen. One is that caution is needed when modifying questionnaires for study populations: do not allow stereotypes to drive the instrument design. I once participated in a meeting to select a questionnaire to assess physical activity levels in a lower-income Hispanic population. A fellow researcher stated that we did not need a category for golf, since low-income Hispanic people do not play golf. In fact, however, if you drive around lower-to-middle income neighborhoods in Tucson, Arizona, you will find driving ranges and courses frequented by low-to-middle-income Mexican Americans. Do not judge your population without doing some research first.

Two, determine whether the modifications you are making to assessment tools are truly ethnic differences or are socioeconomic differences. One way to distinguish between ethnic differences and socioeconomic differences is to question whether the activities that are added or dropped are activities that a particular ethnic group never practices, regardless of economic conditions. In the golf example, as far as I know there is not a religious or cultural taboo against Hispanics playing golf; the presence of numerous Hispanic professional golfers proves this point. On the other hand, golf is a relatively expensive sport, and therefore finances limit who can play.

Three, many tools have been designed for urban dwellers. If you are working in a rural environment, many moderate-to-high-level activities may be missed, such as chopping wood. Unfortunately the design of a culturally appropriate questionnaire takes time, but if that time is invested, you can feel more comfortable about your results.

SUMMARY AND CONCLUSIONS

This paper raises several issues. First, cancer is a leading cause of death for U.S. Hispanics populations, and there is a definite need for research into the behavioral and environmental risk factors. Genetics alone can not account for the differences in incidence rates between non-Hispanic whites and Hispanics, as can be seen by the different incidence rate of colon cancer of Mexicans and Mexican Americans. The heterogeneity of the Hispanic population in the United States alone dispels the notion that all U.S. Hispanic groups can be lumped together to explain lower incidence rates. The regional differences discussed by Trapido et al. (1995) make this very clear.

Second, physical inactivity has been strongly linked with colon cancer in non-Hispanic whites. Breast cancer risk may be reduced for individuals participating in high levels of physical activity during adolescence and early adulthood, but the evidence is still inconclusive. In light of the relationship between physical activity and these cancers, it is important to note that the results of national surveys indicate that in general, U.S. Hispanic populations are less active than non-Hispanic whites. Based on the results of these surveys and previous research on the relationship between physical activity and cancer, one would expect U.S. Hispanic populations to have higher incidence rates of these cancers, not lower. Of course, there are other risk factors involved in these cancers, including genetic, dietary, and smoking history. It may be that the risk is low enough for this population that physical inactivity does not significantly increase risk. Thus the question: Is there a relationship between physical activity and colon or breast cancer risk in U.S. Hispanic populations? Studies looking at the relationships between physical activity and cancer have focused on middle-to-upper-class non-Hispanic whites. While studies may have included individuals with Hispanic ancestry, none has looked at the relationship by ethnicity. It is also expected, based on lower incidence rates, that it is more difficult for research studies to find and enroll eligible Hispanics.

Third, before large studies can be conducted, culturally sensitive physical-activity assessment tools need to be developed, or questions need to be tested in existing tools. Few instruments have been validated in Hispanic populations, much less in different regions of the United States or differing socioeconomic groups. It is important to make sure that the tools have been validated in the target population. If this is not possible, instruments must be pilot-tested within the community they will be used. This should be done even if a tool has been validated.

In order to look at the relationship between physical activity and cancer, assessment tools need to be adapted to reflect adequately the activities of targeted groups. Populations may seem sedentary if key elements of their lifestyles are excluded. In addition, in order to design a questionnaire that is appropriate for generic cancer research, a wide variety of questions is necessary unless you are sure of the biological cause that would link physical activity to the particular cancer.

In summation, little cancer prevention research has focused on physical activity and U.S. Hispanic populations. Methods of assessment need to be altered to incorporate activities that may be ethnically or socioeconomically specific, but caution must also be taken not to exclude activities simply because they do not fit stereotypical notions of a group.

NOTES

1.   For the purpose of this paper, "Hispanic" is defined as Mexican Americans, Puerto Ricans, Cuban Americans, Central Americans, South Americans, and people from other Spanish-speaking Caribbean countries, currently living in the United States. Data sources tend not to differentiate specific ethnic groups when citing cancer risk. The author wishes to emphasize that interethnic variation exists within this category of "Hispanic."

LITERATURE CITED

Albanes, D., A. Blair, and P. R. Taylor. 1989. Physical activity and risk of cancer in the NHANES I population. *American Journal of Public Health* 79:744–750. American Cancer Society. 1994. *Cancer Facts & Figures—1994.* Atlanta.
—. 1997. *Cancer Facts & Figures—1997.* Atlanta.
—. 1998. *Choices for good health: Guidelines for diet, nutrition, and cancer prevention.* 98–500M– no. 2089cc. Atlanta.
Arbman, G., O. Axelson, M. Fredriksson, E. Nilsson, and R. Sjodahl. 1993. Do occupational factors influence the risk of colon and rectal cancer in different ways? *Cancer* 72:2543–2549.
Baecke, J. A. H., J. Burema, and J. E. R Fritjers. 1982. A short questionnaire for the measurement of habitual physical activity in epidemiological studies. *American Journal of Clinical Nutrition* 36:936–942.
Benito, E., A. Obrador, A. Stiggelbout, F. Bosch, M. Mulet, N. Munoz, and J. Kaldor. 1990. A population-based case-control study of colorectal cancer in Majorca: I. dietary factors. *International Journal of Cancer* 45:69–76.
Bernstein, L., B. E. Henderson, R. Hanisch, J. Sullivan-Halley, and R. K. Ross. 1994. Physical exercise and reduced risk of breast cancer in young women. *Journal of the National Cancer Institute* 86:1403–1408.
Bouchard, C. A., A. Tremblay, C. LeBlanc, G. Lortie, R. Sauard, and G. Therialt. 1983. A method to assess energy expenditure in children and adults. *American Journal of Clinical Nutrition* 37:461–467.
Brooks, G. A., and T. D. Fahey. 1985. *Exercise Physiology: Human bioenergetics and its application.* New York: Macmillan.

Calfas, K. J., B. J. Long, J. F. Sallis, W. J. Wooten, M. Pratt, and K. Patrick. 1996. A controlled trial of the physician counseling to promote the adoption of physical activity. *Preventive Medicine* 25:225–233.

Caspersen, C. J., B. P. M. Bloemberg, W. H. M. Saris, R. K. Merritt, and D. Kromhout. 1991. The prevalence of selected physical activities and their relation with coronary heart disease risk factors in elderly men: The Zutphen study. *American Journal of Epidemiology* 133:1078–1092.

DiPietro, L., C. J. Caspersen, A. M. Ostfeld, and E. R. Nadel. 1993. A survey for assessing physical activity among older adults. *Medicine and Science in Sports and Exercise* 25:628–642.

Dorgan, J. F., C. Brown, M. Barrett, G. L. Splansky, B. E. Kreger, R. B. D'Agostino, D. Albanes, and A. Schatzkin. 1994. Physical activity and risk of breast cancer in the Framingham heart study. *American Journal of Epidemiology* 1139:662–669.

Dosemeci, M., R. B. Hayes, R. Vetter, R. N. Hoover, M. Tucker, K. Engin, M. Unsal, and A. Blair. 1993. Occupational physical activity, socioeconomic status, and risks of 15 cancer sites in Turkey. *Cancer Causes and Control* 4:313–321.

Fredriksson, M., N. O. Bengtsson, L. Hardell, and O. Axelson. 1989. Colon cancer, physical activity, and occupational exposures. A case-control study. *Cancer* 63:1838–1842.

Garcia-Palmieri, M. R. R., J. Costas, M. Cruz-Vidal, P. D. Sorlie, and R. J. Avlik. 1982. Increased physical activity: a protective factor against heart attacks in Puerto Rico. *American Journal of Cardiology* 50:749–755.

Godin, G., and R. J. Shephard. 1985. A simple method to assess exercise behavior in the community. *Canadian Journal of Applied Sport Science* 10:141–146.

Hsing, A. W., J. K. McLaughlin, W. Zheng, Y. T. Gao, and W. J. Blot. 1994. Occupation, physical activity, and risk of prostate cancer in Shanghai, People's Republic of China. *Cancer Causes and Control* 5:136–140.

Jacobs, D. R., Jr., L. P. Hahn, W. L. Haskell, P. Pirie, and S. Sidney. 1989. Validity and reliability of short physical activity history: Cardia and the Minnesota heart health program. *Journal of Cardiopulmonary Rehabilitation* 9:449–459.

Kohl, H. W., S. N. Blair, J. Paffenbarger, C. A. Macera, and J. J. Kronenfeld. 1988. A mail survey of physical activity habits as related to measures of fitness. *American Journal of Epidemiology* 127:1228–1239.

Kono, S., K. Shinchi, N. Ikeda, F. Yanai, and K. Imanishi. 1991. Physical activity, dietary habits and ademnomatous polyps of the sigmoid colon: A study of self-defense officials in Japan. *Journal of Clinical Epidemiology* 44(11):1255–1261.

Kriska, A .M., and P. H. Bennett. 1992. An epidemiological perspective of the relationship between physical activity and NIDDM: From activity assessment to intervention. *Diabetes Metabolism Review* 8:355–372.

Kriska, A. M., W. C. Knowler, R. E. LaPorte, A. L. Drash, R. R. Wing, S. N. Blair, P. H. Bennett, and L. H. Kuller. 1990. Development of questionnaire to examine relationship of physical activity and diabetes in Pima Indians. *Diabetes Care* 13:401–411.

Kune, G. A., S. Kune, and L. F. Watson. 1990. Body weight and physical activity as predictors of colorectal cancer risk. *Nutrition and Cancer* 13:9–17.

Lakka, T. A., and J. T. Salonen. 1992. Physical activity and serum lipids: A cross-sectional population study in eastern Finnish men. *American Journal of Epidemiology* 136:806–818.

Lee, H., L. Gourley, S. Duffy, J. Esteve, J. Lee, and N. Day. 1989. Colorectal cancer and diet in an Asian population: A case-control study among Singapore Chinese. *International Journal of Cancer* 43:1007–1016.

Lee, I. M., R. S. Paffenberger, Jr., and C. Hsieh. 1991. Physical activity and risk of developing colorectal cancer among college alumni. *Journal of the National Cancer Institute* 83:1324–1329.

Marcus, B. H., P. M. Dubbert, A. C. King, and B. M. Pinto. 1995. Physical activity in women: Current status and future directions. In *The psychology of women's health: Progress and challenges in research and application*, ed. A. Stanton and S. Gallant, 349-379. Washington, DC: American Psychological Association.

Marcus, P. M., P. A. Newcomb, and B. E. Storer. 1994. Early adulthood physical activity and colon cancer risk among Wisconsin women. *Cancer Epidemiology, Biomarkers and Prevention* 3:641–644.

Martinez, M. E., E. Giovannucci, D. Spiegelmen, D. J. Hunter, W. C. Willett, and G. A. Colditz. 1997. Leisure-time physical activity, body size, and colon cancer in women. Nurses' Health Study Research Group. *Journal of the National Cancer Institute* 89:948–955.

Miller, B. A., L. N. Kolonel, L. Bernstein, J. L. Young, Jr., G. M. Swanson, D. West, C. R. Key, J. M. Liff, C. S. Glover, G. A. Alexander, et al., eds. 1996. *Racial/ethnic patterns of cancer in the United States, 1988–1992*. NIH Pub. no. 96–4104. Bethesda: National Cancer Institute.

Montoye, H. J. 1971. Estimation of habitual physical activity by questionnaire and interview. *American Journal of Clinical Nutrition* 24:1113–1118.

Montoye, H. J., H. C. G. Kemper, W. H. M. Saris, and R. A. Washburn. 1996. *Measuring physical activity and energy expenditure*. Champaign, IL: Human Kinetics.

Nader, P. R., D. E. Sellers, C. C. Johnson, C. L. Perry, E. J. Stone, K. C. Cook, J. Bebchuk, and R. V. Luepker. 1996. The effect of adult participation in a school-based family intervention to improve children's diet and physical activity: The child and adolescent trial for cardiovascular health. *Preventive Medicine* 25:455–464.

Paffenbarger, R. S., R. T. Hyde, and A. L. Wing. 1987. Physical activity and incidence of cancer in diverse populations: A preliminary report. *American Journal of Clinical Nutrition* 45:312–317.

Paffenbarger, R. S., R. T. Hyde, A. L. Wing, I. M. Lee, D. L. Jung, and J. B. Kampert. 1993. The association of changes in physical-activity level and other lifestyle characteristics with mortality among men. *New England Journal of Medicine* 328(8):538–545.

Paffenbarger, R. S., A. L. Wing, and R. T. Hyde. 1978. Physical activity as an index of heart attack risk in college alumni. *American Journal of Epidemiology* 108:161–175.

Pereira, M. A., S. J. Fitzgerald, E. W. Gregg, M. L. Joswiak, W. J. Ryan, R. R. Suminski, A. C. Utter, and M. Zmuda. 1997. A collection of physical activity questionnaires for health-related research. *Medicine and Science in Sports and Exercise* 29:Supplement.

Perry, C. L., E. J. Stone, G. S. Parcel, R. C. Ellison, P. R. Nader, L. S. Webber, and R. V. Luepker. 1990. School-based cardiovascular health promotion: The child and adolescent trial for cardiovascular health (CATCH). *Journal of School Health* 60:406–413.

Ramirez, A. G., R. Villarreal, L. Suarez, and E. T. Flores. 1995. The emerging Hispanic population: A foundation for cancer prevention and control. *Journal of the National Cancer Institute Monograph* 18:1–9.

Rauh, M. J. D., M. F. Hovell, C. R. Hofstetter, J. F. Sallis, and A. Gleghorn. 1992. Reliability and validity of self-reported physical activity in Latinos. *International Journal of Epidemiology* 21:966–971.

Sallis, J. F., M. J. Buono, J. J. Roby, F. G. Micale, and J. A Nelson. 1993. Seven-day recall and other physical activity self-reports in children and adolescents. *Medicine and Science in Sports and Exercise* 25:99–108.

Salonen, J. T., and T. Lakka. 1987 Assessment of physical activity in population studies: Validity and consistency of the methods in the Kuopio ischaemic heart disease risk factor study. *Scandinavian Journal of Sports Science* 9:89–95.

Savitz, D. A. 1986. Changes in Spanish surname cancer rates relative to other whites, Denver area, 1969–71 to 1979–81. *American Journal of Public Health* 76:1210–1215.

Shea, S., A. D. Stein, R. Lantigua, and C. E. Basch. 1991. Reliability of the behavioral risk factor survey in a triethnic population. *American Journal of Epidemiology* 133:489–500.

Shu, X. O., M. C. Hatch, W. Zheng, Y. T. Gao, and L. A. Brinton. 1993. Physical activity and risk of endometrial cancer. *Epidemiology* 4:342–349.

Sidney S., Jr., W. L. Haskell, M. A. Armstrong, A. Dimicco, A. Oberman, P. J. Savage, M. L. Slattery, B. Sternfeld, and L. V. Horn. 1991. Comparison of two methods of assessing physical activity in the coronary artery risk development in young adults (CARDIA) study. *American Journal of Epidemiology* 133:1231–1245.

Slattery, M. L., N. Abd-Elghany, R. Kerber, and M. C. Schumacher. 1990. Physical activity and colon cancer: A comparison of various indicators of physical activity to evaluate the association. *Epidemiology* 1:481–485.

Stukonis, M., and R. Doll. 1969. Gastric cancer in man and physical activity at work. *International Journal of Cancer* 4:248–254.

Taylor, H. L., Jr., B. Schucker, J. Knudsen, A. S. Leon, and G. Debaker. 1978. A questionnaire for the assessment of leisure time physical activity. *Journal of Chronic Disease* 31:741–755.

Thun, M., E. Calle, M. Namboodiri, W. Flanders, R. Coates, T. Byers, P. Boffetta, L. Garfinkel, and C. J. Heath. 1992. Risk factors for fatal colon cancer in a large prospective study. *Journal of National Cancer Institute*: 1491–1500.

Thune, I., T. Brenn, E. Lund, and M. Gaard. 1997. Physical activity and the risk of breast cancer. *New England Journal of Medicine* 336:1269–1275.

Trapido, E. J., R. B. Valdez, J. L. Obeso, N. Strickman-Stein, A. Rotger, and E. J. Pérez-Stable. 1995. Epidemiology of cancer among Hispanics in the United States. *Journal of the National Cancer Institute Monographs* 18:17–27.

U.S. Department of Health and Human Services. 1996. *Physical activity and health: A report of the Surgeon General.* Atlanta: Centers for Disease Control and Prevention, National Center for Chronic Disease Prevention and Promotion, International Medical Publishing.

Vena, J. E., S. Graham, M. Zielezny, J. Brasure, and M. K. Swanson. 1987. Occupational exercise and risk of cancer. *American Jounral of Clinical Nutrition* 45:318–327.

Vetter, R., M. Dosemeci, A. Blair, S. Wacholder, M. Unsal, K. Engin, and J. F. Fraumeni, Jr. 1992. Occupational physical activity and colon cancer risk in Turkey. *European Journal of Epidemiology* 8:845–850.

Vineis, P., G. Ciccone, and A. Magnino. 1993. Asbestos exposure, physical activity and colon cancer: A case-control study. *Tumori* 79:301–303.

Washburn, R. A., K. W. Smith, A. M. Jette, and C. A. Janney. 1993. The physical activity scale for the elderly (PASE): Development and evaluation. *Journal of Clinical Epidemiology* 46:153–162.

Zheng, W., X. O. Shu, J. K. McLaughlin, W. H. Chow, Y. T. Gao, and W. J. Blot. 1993. Occupational physical activity and the incidence of cancer of the breast, corpus uteri, and the ovary in Shanghai. *Cancer* 71:3620–3624.

Chapter 15

Diet-Cancer Associations: Insights Offered by Native Americans

Nicolette I. Teufel

In the United States in the 1970s, interest in the role played by diet in the promotion or suppression of cancer became a part of the national goal of "winning the war against cancer." In 1971, the National Cancer Institute (NCI) received a congressional mandate to investigate the relationship between nutrition and cancer. In 1982, the U.S. National Academy of Sciences (NAS), commissioned by NCI, published *Diet, Nutrition and Cancer* (NAS 1982). In 1997, the World Cancer Research Fund (WCRF) and the American Institute for Cancer Research (AICR) published *Food, Nutrition and the Prevention of Cancer: A Global Perspective* (WCRF/AICR 1997). This 1997 review offered an evaluation of the scientific literature linking foods, nutrition, food preparation, dietary patterns, and related factors with the risk of human cancers worldwide, and also a series of dietary recommendations suitable for all societies to reduce the risk of cancer (WCRF/AICR 1997, 6).

The purpose of this chapter is to discuss carcinogenesis as related to dietary factors, to provide a synopsis of proposed diet-cancer associations, and to apply this information to a review of the dietary patterns and cancer incidence rates reported for Native Americans living in the Southwest. The latter exercise will explore "the fit" between national epidemiological patterns and culture-specific populations. The argument is made that "a lack of fit" should not be ignored, that it could provide tremendous insight into limitations of the scientific process, or into unique conditions that might increase or decrease the risk of cancer in specific populations.

DIET AND THE CANCER PROCESS

Cancer is characterized by disordered and excessive cell replication. Carcinogens are agents that alter a cell's genetic code, thereby promoting cancerous growth. Exposure to carcinogens is influenced by environmental quality (e.g., exposure to asbestos, DDT), behavior (e.g., tobacco use, food preparation and storage techniques, food choices, alcohol consumption, and occupation), and the normal process of cell metabolism. Cell metabolism creates oxygen radicals, molecules that are electron deficient. These oxygen radicals can act as carcinogens, damaging genetic material. Generally, this damage is repaired as a regular part of maintenance activities; if the damage is not repaired, carcinogenesis can be initiated.

Dietary components can both protect against and promote carcinogenesis. Table 15.1 provides a summary of the diet and cancer associations, by cancer site (WCRF/AICR 1997).

DIET AND THE PROMOTION OF CARCINOGENESIS

Food Behavior

Some dietary compounds, generally associated with the handling, preparation, and storage of foods, are carcinogenic (see Table 15.2). Salt and foods that have been salted, pickled (soaked in a salty brine), cured, or smoked, particularly meats and fish, have been associated with an increased risk of cancers of the digestive tract (e.g., larynx, nasopharynx, esophagus, stomach, colon, and rectum) (Nomura et al. 1990; Lu et al. 1991; Kneller et al. 1991; Zheng et al. 1992; WCRF/AICR 1997). The WCRF/AICR (1997) report concludes that high levels of heterocyclic amines found in grilled and barbecued meats and fish cooked at high temperatures increase the risk of stomach, colon, and rectal cancer. Preserving foods by drying may also yield dietary carcinogens. For example, some dried food plants have been found to contain carcinogenic N-nitroso compounds (WCRF/AICR 1997).

Meal frequency has been proposed as a risk factor for some cancers, particularly colon cancer (Potter and McMichael 1986; LaVecchia et al. 1988; Gerhardsson de Verdier and Longnecker 1992). Eating bouts increase bile excretion and trigger the gastro-ileal reflex. Bile acids, potentially carcinogenic to colon cells, may enter the colon with the increased reflex action and initiate chromosomal damage. A small increase (10% to 20%) in risk is associated with each daily eating occasion (WCRF/AICR 1997).

Nutrients

If genetic damage has been initiated, nutrients can promote carcinogenic cell growth. Excessive intakes of fat, animal protein, refined starches, sugars, or energy (calories) have been shown to enhance cell proliferation (Poirier et al.

1986; Kritchevsky and Klurfeld 1987; Pariza 1987; Wattenberg 1992; LaVecchia et al. 1993) and have been associated with cancers of the breast, colon, prostate, pancreas, rectum, gallbladder, and endometrium (Armstrong and Doll 1975; WCRF/AICR 1997) (see Table 15.3).

Alcohol may act as a cocarcinogen or a promoting agent in carcinogenesis. Mechanisms explaining alcohol's carcinogenic effect include: (1) alteration of the mucosal cells of the upper respiratory tract, the digestive tract, the colon, and the rectum; (2) alcohol-induced nutrient deficiencies, with alcohol replacing potentially protective micronutrient-dense foods; (3) damage to liver-cell genetic material; and (4) changes in estrogen levels, promoting hormone-related cancers. Alcohol intake has been identified as a potential risk factor for cancers of the mouth, pharynx, nasopharynx, larynx, esophagus, breast, liver, colon, and rectum (WCRF/AICR 1997).

DIET AND THE SUPPRESSION OF CARCINOGENESIS

A restriction in total energy intake has been shown to suppress gene activity associated with the formation of spontaneous tumors (Hursting et al. 1994). Evidence for the protective effect of low energy intake is strongest for pancreatic cancer (Tannenbaum 1959; Pariza 1987) and prostate cancer (Rohan et al. 1995).

Vitamins and Minerals

Several dietary compounds, found predominantly in fruits and vegetables, can inhibit carcinogenesis (Table 15.4). Carotenoids, vitamins C and E, and selenium are antioxidants, capable of deactivating or scavenging oxygen radicals (electron-deficient molecules) and protecting cell membranes and genetic material from potentially carcinogenic activity (Peto et al. 1981). These same micronutrients may play a role in the body's defense against carcinogenesis, via their support of immune function. Vitamin A, derived from carotenoids, is essential to normal cell growth, maintenance, and differentiation; it may play a role in suppressing cancer development.

Carotenoids are yellow, orange, and red pigments synthesized by plants. Many dark green foods, such as parsely, broccoli, and green beans, are rich in carotenoids but the green pigment (chlorophyll) masks the bright carotenoid color. Carotenoids are abundant in carrots, sweet potatoes, pumpkins, and other orange and yellow squashes, peaches, apricots, oranges, cantaloupe, watermelon, tomatoes, and red peppers.

Vitamin C, associated with citrus fruits, is also present in milk, broccoli, cabbage, peppers, tomatoes, pumpkins, fresh potatoes, bananas, strawberries, melons, and fortified fruit drinks. Vitamin E is present in vegetable oils, including margarine, mayonnaise, and shortening, as well as in whole grains, nuts, seeds, and dark green leafy vegetables.

Selenium has been shown to enhance immune function, decrease the mutagenic effect of carcinogens, and suppress cancer cell proliferation. Selenium has been associated with a decreased risk of lung and prostate cancer. Selenium is found in whole grains, seeds, and seafood.

Folate or folic acid is involved in the replication and maintenance of genetic material (purines and pyrimidines). Folate deficiencies have been associated with an increased risk of genetic abnormalities. Folate is abundant in whole grains, legumes, dark green leafy vegetables, and liver.

Dietary Fiber

High fiber diets have been linked to a possibly decreased risk of breast, stomach, pancreatic, colon, and rectal cancer (WCRF/AICR 1997). Dietary fiber is available primarily in whole grains, fruits, and vegetables. Fiber's protective mechansims include dilution of carcinogenic agents, absorption and elimination of carcinogens, and reduction of tissue-carcinogen contact.

Bioactive Compounds

Other nonnutritive, bioactive compounds obtained through the diet have also been associated with a reduced risk of cancer or have been shown to play a role in cancer protection. Protease inhibitors, found in whole grains, seeds, and legumes (e.g., kidney beans, chickpeas, pinto beans), form compounds that block the enzyme protease. Protease plays a role in the invasive action of malignant cancer cells.

Limonene, a trepenoid and a major component of the oil in citrus fruit peel, may provide cancer protection by inducing glutathione transferases, enzymes shown to inhibit tumor formation (Wattenberg 1983; Elson and Yu 1994). Dietary exposure to limonene is usually as a flavoring agent in nonalcoholic beverages, ice cream, gelatins, puddings, baked goods, and chewing gum.

Flavonoids, found in fruits (predominantly berries, tomatoes, and citrus fruits), vegetables (predominantly potatoes, broccoli, and dark greens), coffee, tea, cola, and alcoholic beverages, have been shown to function as antioxidants, deactivating oxygen radicals.

Isoflavones and lignans are heterocyclic phenols and heterocyclic phenol precursors, respectively. These compounds, which occur primarily in seeds, berries containing seeds, whole grains, soybeans, and possibly other legumes, act as phytoestrogens, forming hormonelike compounds after digestion. Hormones, such as estrogen, have been shown to play a promotional role in carcinogenesis, particularly in breast cancer. Phytoestrogens may have a protective effect, by binding to estrogen receptors and blocking the attachment of more potent estrogens, which may stimulate carcinogenesis.

Polyphenol extracts of green tea have been shown to have an anticarcinogenic effect in animals. Case-control studies in Japan (Kono et al. 1988; Kato et al. 1990;) and China (Yu et al. 1995) suggest that green tea can have a protective effect relative to stomach cancer. The proposed mechanism of protection is suppression of carcinogenesis upon exposure to carcinogens.

Food Behaviors

Food behaviors, other than food choice, may reduce cancer risk. Access to refrigeration may decrease cancer risk, by promoting year-round fruit and vegetable consumption, reducing reliance on food preservation techniques like salting, curing, and smoking, and delaying food spoilage (minimizing exposure to aflatoxins and N-nitroso compounds). Access to gas and electric cooking facilities may reduce exposure to heterocyclic amines, carcinogens formed in meats cooked at high temperatures and over open flames.

NATIVE AMERICANS, DIET AND CANCER: AN EPIDEMIOLOGICAL ENIGMA OR A TEST OF DIET-CANCER HYPOTHESES?

Dietary surveys collected with Native Americans over the past fifteen years present a diet high in fat, energy, and in some instances alcohol, and low in fiber and micronutrient-dense fruits and vegetables. These dietary patterns are associated with an increased risk of cancer at multiple sites. Yet for many diet-related cancers, Native Americans actually have lower cancer incidence rates than other ethnic groups in the United Stated (see Table 15.1). A review of traditional and contemporary dietary practices of Native Americans living in the Southwest and a critical examination of dietary assessment methods are presented to offer insight into this apparent paradox.

Dietary Intake among Southwest Native Americans

Table 15.5 compares anthropometric data, dietary characteristics, and select mean dietary intakes of Native American women representing four tribes located in the southwestern United States—the Hualapai, the Apache, the Pima, and the Navajo. All data presented were collected between 1985 and 1995 from participants living in these reservation communities. Two factors influenced the selection of these data: (1) reports included micronutrient information relevant to cancer promotion or suppression; and (2) these tribes are culturally distinct, providing a diverse picture of the dietary patterns in this geographic region.

Linguistically and genetically, the Apache and Navajo are related, descendants of nomadic Athabascan-speaking peoples who migrated into the Southwest from western Canada prior to A.D. 1500. The Hualapai and Pima are not closely related to each other or to the Athabascan-speaking groups. The Hualapai and Pima are Yuman and Piman-speaking peoples, respectively, and prehistoric roots in the Southwest are documented for both.

Some surveys did not include data from men; consequently only women's intake from the four tribes is presented, to allow a uniform comparison. The Hualapai data are the result of twenty-four-hour dietary recalls collected for seven consecutive days from a twenty-eight-woman volunteer sample (196 total dietary recalls). The Apache data represent twenty-four-hour dietary recalls collected for six random days (four weekdays and two weekend days) from a twenty-seven-woman volunteer sample (162 total dietary recalls). The Pima and Navajo data are derived from single twenty-four-hour dietary recalls collected from 273 women (volunteer sample) and 225 women (random sample), respectively. All data were collected via face-to-face interviews by trained native and nonnative interviewers. Standard deviations are greater in the samples composed of multiple-day records collected from a few women than in the single-day records collected from a larger number of women. In a cross-sample comparison, dietary variation presented by intra-individual variation is greater than for inter-individual variation.

The relative contribution of fat, carbohydrate, and protein in total energy intake is presented to allow a comparison to the WCRF/AICR recommendations. The macronutrient composition of the women's diets is similar; percentage of energy from alcohol, however, is not similar. This dissimilarity may be an artifact of the difficulty in collecting accurate alcohol-intake data. Nondietary reports of alcohol consumption suggest that intakes do not vary substantially by tribe (Kunitz et al. 1979; Everett 1980; Topper 1980; Waddell and Everett 1980; May 1982; May et al. 1983; Teufel 1994).

Intertribal dietary similarities are created by a shared low mean income, reliance on federal food assistance programs (e.g., the USDA Food Commodity Program; the Women, Infants and Children (WIC) Food Assistance Program; and the Elderly Nutrition Program), and similar cooking techniques. The most frequently selected foods from the USDA Food Commodity Program include white flour, yellow cornmeal, butter, vegetable oil, rice, fortified fruit drinks, and canned vegetables, fruits, and meats. The WIC Food Assistance Program provides vouchers for the purchase of specific nutrient-dense foods such as milk, cheese, and fortified cereals. Participation in the USDA Food Commodity Program and the WIC Food Assistance Program contributes to the comparably high intakes of protein (cheese and milk) and vitamin E (yellow cornmeal, butter, and vegetable oils).

High body mass indices reported for three of the four samples indicate that caloric intake is greater than caloric expenditure. WCRF/AICR does not provide a recommended range for energy intake, since appropriate energy intake is variable, relative to level of energy expenditure. High energy intake coupled with increasingly sedentary behavior has been reported previously among indigenous populations subjected to such social changes as adapting to new foods and new occupations introduced by nonnatives (Teufel 1999).

The following generalized food source information was provided in conjunction with the dietary reports cited in Table 15.5. In all four tribes, potatoes, white flour, and soft drinks are the predominant sources of carbohydrates. Beef, beans, eggs, and canned meat (e.g., corned beef and Spam[tm]) are the predominant sources of protein. Cooking fats and oils (including lard and butter) are the predominant sources of dietary fat. The primary source of dietary fiber is legumes. Fortified fruits drinks (e.g., Hi-C[tm] and Tang[tm]) make the greatest contribution to total vitamin C intake.

Despite general similarities, intertribal diversity should not be ignored. Differences in vitamin C, dietary fiber, and to a lesser degree protein can be attributed in part to cultural preferences and different access to food stores. The small markets or trading posts in many reservation communities stock only a limited supply of produce. The Hualapai and portions of the Apache and Navajo reservations are more than fifty miles from well-stocked supermarkets that offer a range of fresh produce. In these communities, household food purchasing is characterized by a greater reliance on small markets and a tendency to choose foods having a long shelf life (e.g., potatoes and canned foods). Fresh fruits and vegetables, rich sources of vitamin C, carotenoids, and dietary fiber, are less frequently consumed in these communities. For some Navajo this effect may not be evident, as larger Navajo communities (e.g., Kayenta, Window Rock, and Tuba City) have supermarkets, with wide selections of fresh produce. Most Pima communities are less than thirty miles from supermarkets, on and off the reservation in Casa Grande, or in communities outside of Phoenix. Different access to fresh produce may explain differences in intakes of vitamin C and fiber.

The percentages and means reported in Table 15.5 reflect a diet low in fruits and vegetables and high in meat and fat. These dietary behaviors have been associated with an increased risk of cancer. Yet at many diet-related cancer sites, Native Americans do not suffer cancer incidence rates comparable to that of the United States, all races. This paradox suggests that other factors may be confounding the diet-cancer associations.

Possible explanations for the observed inconsistencies between Southwest Native American dietary behaviors and cancer incidence rates are: (1) a delayed generational effect of dietary change; (2) absence of confounding factors (e.g., low prevalence of smoking in Southwest Native Americans, which may influence more than lung cancer rates); (3) genetic differences in susceptibility to specific cancers (Morris et al. 1978; Sievers and Fisher 1983; Sorem 1985); (4) underreporting of national and international studies demonstrating no diet-cancer associations (thus magnifying the importance of studies demonstrating significant diet-cancer associations); and (5) inadequate assessment of culturally distinct dietary behaviors. The remainder of this chapter will explore the last proposed explanation. It will address the ability of dietary assessment methods frequently employed to record dietary behaviors and to estimate nutrient intake in culturally distinct populations.

HUMAN BEHAVIOR AND DIETARY ASSESSMENT METHODS

Many diet-disease associations have been proposed by epidemiological studies. Nutritional epidemiologists typically use twenty-four-hour dietary recalls or food-frequency questionnaires to assess population patterns of nutrient intake.

In general, dietary assessment methods were developed by Europeans or Euro-Americans, and they work best in the collection of European/American-type diets and dietary behaviors. For example, if consumption of nuts and seeds is reported, they assume that the shells were not eaten (a Euro-American behavior). Yet in some cultural settings, particularly in the consumption of very-high-fat or soft-shelled nuts and seeds, the hulls may be eaten (Teufel 1989). The interviewee may not think to report shell consumption, thinking it is "normal" or "assumed" behavior; the interviewer assumes no shell consumption, and a significant intake of fiber is lost from the total dietary record. Data collectors not from the specific cultural group may not be aware of distinct behaviors and may fail to ask appropriate questions. If data collectors are aware of such behaviors but are not sure how to record them on standardized data collection forms, nutrients may be underrepresented in calculations of total dietary intake.

The following examples of food behaviors practiced by some Southwest Native Americans are provided to suggest that micronutrient intakes may be greater than those reported. These case studies illustrate potential inadequacies of dietary assessment methods and are offered to encourage a reexamination of methodology. Any method designed to evaluate human behavior, such as food choice and preparation, must be subjected to constant scrutiny to assess the cultural competency of the technique (Teufel 1997). The assumptions, inherent to any data collection method developed out of one culture, may not be applicable or appropriate in another culture.

CASE STUDIES

Case Study #1: Carotenoids, Vitamin C, Folate, Fiber, and Wild Plant Foods

Many Southwest Native Americans still consume wild plant foods. Availability of these foods is seasonal, but many households dry or (more recently) freeze foods for occasional consumption throughout the year. Families collect wild greens or spinach, cactus fruits and pads, agave cores and fruits, wild nuts, and a variety of cooking herbs. Depending on the ecozone, season, and tribe, wild greens may include pigweed (Amaranthus spp.), lambsquarters (Chenopodium spp.), Indian spinach (Monolepis nuttaliana), saltbush (Atriplex spp.), purslane (Portulaca oleracea), or beeweed (Cleome integrifolia or Peritoma serulatum). Compared to domesticated spinach, many of these greens are higher in iron, calcium, vitamin C, carotenoids, and fiber and are similar in folate (Kuhnlein et al. 1979; Wolfe et al. 1985; Smith et al. 1993; Teufel 1998). When interviewed, a respondent may believe that the interviewer is not familiar with wild greens or may think the consumption inappropriate relative to the interviewer's cultural values. In this case, wild greens may be simply reported as spinach. Even if the data collector *is* familiar with wild greens, the food may still get recorded as spinach—to minimize confusion for nonnative nutritionists or data entry personnel, or to provide an analog, as many wild foods are not in the standard nutrient databases used in dietary analysis programs. As a result of this substitution, the respondent does not get credit for significant intakes of micronutrients.

Case Study #2: Vitamin E, Protease Inhibitors, and Sunflower Seeds

Nuts and seeds are good sources of vitamin E and protease inhibitors. In the Southwest, some Native Americans consume large quantities of sunflower seeds. Sunflower seeds are frequently carried around in a pocket or kept in an easily accessible place and consumed throughout the day. Generally, they are not reported in dietary surveys. To interviewees, the nutrient contribution of sunflower seeds seems trivial, and their consumption is inadvertently omitted. If the interviewer is not alerted to probe for sunflower seeds, a potential source of vitamin E and protease inhibitors will be missed.

In a high school–based health education program, some young Native American males were regularly consuming 20,000µg/day of vitamin E (>110% of the WCRF/AICR recommendation for vitamin E intake—see Table 15.1), primarily in sunflower seeds. The impact of large intakes of potentially cancer protective agents has not been evaluated and may offer a clue to understanding the diet-cancer paradox proposed for Native Americans.

Case Study #3: Limonene and Lemons

Limonene, a bioactive compound found primarily in citrus fruits, has been associated with a reduced risk of digestive cancers, particularly stomach (and potentially colon) cancer. The greatest concentration of limonene is found in the underside of the peel in citrus fruits. In the Southwest, Native Americans, particularly children and adolescents, eat lemons as snacks. When lemons have been eaten and the fruit consumed, kids scrape the inside of the peel with their teeth and on occasion chew the peel. Most often the consumption of lemons as snacks is not reported. When interviewees are asked about snacks, generally potato chips and tortilla chips are mentioned. If citrus consumption is recorded, the assumption is that only the fruit and juice are consumed. Yet Native Americans may have an increased exposure to limonene, afforded by the habit of eating or scraping the peel. This exposure is greatest in children and adolescents, for whom the impact of dietary prevention might be the greatest. Could this association help explain Native Americans' reduced risk of colon cancer, despite reportedly low intakes of fruits and vegetables?

OTHER ASSESSMENT ISSUES

Other factors that may magnify the effect of questions and questionnaires not recording culturally distinct behaviors are overtraining local data collectors and overstandardizing the data collection process. Researchers who recognize the potential impact of regional or cultural differences will often hire local data collectors. These data collectors, and sometimes community members, are often asked to review the questions for cultural appropriateness. The primary goal of this exercise is to avoid miscommunication, inadvertent insults, or discussion of inappropriate topics. Native community members, however, are rarely asked what they believe is the cause of the illness being studied or the relationship between certain behaviors, illness, and health. If questions relevant to cultural etiologies are included, the addition is often intended to provide a tally of the percentage of people surveyed who still adhere to cultural traditions and beliefs. The question becomes a measure of acculturation. Often the words "still adhere" are employed in the final report, suggesting that the hold on traditional culture is tenuous and that over time these ideas will fade and the biomedical explanation will prevail.

Standardized data collection processes (questionnaires, guidelines standardizing prompts and probes, etc.) are used in all research settings, including culturally distinct settings. One remedy to enhance the cultural appropriateness of standardized assessment tools is to add culturally relevant questions. The design of questions and of any supplemental guidelines outlining the level of interview interaction (e.g., reading questions aloud, explaining terminology, or exploring other seemingly unrelated behaviors) is often carefully controlled by the researcher, often nonNative. If normal interpersonal interactions are controlled in an attempt to standardize and focus the data-collection process, unspoken assumptions or unreported behaviors may devalue the information collected. As illustrated, if a lemon is recorded as a snack and the assumption is made that only the fruit and juice are consumed, the interviewee will not get "nutrient credit" for portions of the peel. Standardized methods do not ensure accurate information.

Recommendations for avoiding these pitfalls in exploring cancer risks and outcomes in culturally distinct populations include working with local consultants: (1) to ask what they think causes cancer; (2) to share the biomedical objectives of the proposed survey or study; (3) to ask how they would collect the information incorporating the biomedical and local etiological explanations and risk factors; and (4) to collaborate on the modification of standardized methods or the development of new methods. Avoid teaching or overemphasizing the biomedical model. In the United States, people who have been labeled as ethnic minorities are often experts in blending cultural perspectives to yield adaptive behaviors. Their expertise will strengthen the knowledge and relevancy of the survey or study results.

For example, cultural perspectives could be blended in the design of a culture-specific food frequency questionnaire (FFQ). In one particular cultural setting, squash and green beans, when eaten in large quantities, were considered comparable to meat, beans, or other high-protein foods. Standard FFQs place squash and green beans in the fruit and vegetable category and allow only for relatively small serving sizes (one-quarter, one-half, or one cup). Native colleagues suggested eliminating the use of nutrient-based food groups (meats, dairy products, fruits and vegetables, etc.) and categorizing foods by role (e.g., main dishes, snacks, side dishes). This format allowed respondents to think about squash and green beans in the appropriate cultural context (with beans and meat) and to report freely large serving sizes.

CONCLUDING REMARKS

Epidemiological and experimental studies offer increasing evidence of the relationship between diet and cancer. Epidemiological studies depend upon questions and questionnaires to assess food behaviors and nutrient intakes. As illustrated by the three case studies of Southwest Native Americans, dietary assessment methods may not capture culturally distinct food behaviors. If subtle differences in dietary behavior are not recorded, reported nutrient intakes may not accurately predict diet-related disease risks. If generally accepted diet-disease associations are not observed in these culturally distinct settings, these populations may surface as epidemiological enigmas. Findings of no association may be attributed to small sample size, unidentified confounding factors, or genetic differences in disease risk or nutrient metabolism.

This examination of the dietary behaviors of Southwest Native Americans and the low incidence among them of some diet-related cancers challenges epidemiologists and other researchers to review the cultural competency of their data collection methods. A primary goal in questionnaire development is to ensure that the questionnaire designers and respondents have a comparable understanding of the meanings of words. Working toward this goal requires an understanding of the "common ground," the collection of shared assumptions. Questionnaire designers must know how respondents will interpret words and associations and, perhaps more importantly, address the emotional consequences of specific responses.

By the year 2050, greater than 50% of the U.S. population will self-identify as members of cultural groups of non-European ancestry. Questions addressing the cultural relevance and applicability of diet and other behavioral assessment methods are important to understanding not only cancer risks and outcomes but many of the nation's patterns of health and disease.

ACKNOWLEDGMENTS

The author would like to thank members of the Hualapai, Apache, Hopi, and Zuni communities for sharing their time and expertise. Their willingness to work with the author made much of the information and insight offered in this paper possible.

This research was funded in part by NIH/NCI Grant No. CA68460-03.

LITERATURE CITED

Armstrong, B., and Doll, R. 1975. Environmental factors and cancer incidence and mortality in different countries, with special reference to dietary practices. *International Journal of Cancer* 15:617–631.

Ballew, C., L. L. White, K. F. Strauss, L. J. Benson, J. M. Mendlein, and A. H. Mokdad. 1997. Intake of nutrients and food sources of nutrients among the Navajo: Findings from the Navajo health and nutrition survey. *Journal of Nutrition* 127(Suppl.10S):2085S–2093S.

Baquet, C. R. 1992. Cancer research with special populations. Keynote presentation at Cancer in Indian Country: A National Conference, 17 September, sponsored by The Native American Research and Training Center, University of Arizona, College of Medicine, Tucson, Arizona.

Buckley, D. I., R. S. McPherson, C. Q. North, and T. M. Becker. 1992. Dietary micronutrients and cervical dysplasia in southwestern American Indian women. *Nutrition and Cancer* 17(2):179–185.

Burhansstipanov, L., and C. M. Dresser. 1993. *Native American monograph no. 1: Documentation of the cancer research needs of American Indians and Alaska Natives.* NIH Publication No. 93-3603. Washington, DC: National Cancer Institute.

De Giovanni, G. M. 1995. Micronutrient intake values and cervical dysplasia and cancer in Hualapai and Apache Women. Ph.D. Dissertation, University of Arizona, Tucson.

Elson, C. E., and S. G Yu. 1994. The chemoprevention of cancer by mevalonate-derived constituents of fruits and vegetables. *Journal of Nutrition* 124(5):607–614.

Everett, M. W. 1980. Drinking as a measure of proper behavior: The White Mountain Apaches. In *Drinking behavior among southwestern Indians: An anthropological perspective,* ed. J. O. Waddell and M. W. Everett, 148–177. Tucson: University of Arizona Press.

Gerhardsson de Verdier, M., and M. P. Longnecker. 1992. Eating frequency: A neglected risk factor for colon cancer? *Cancer Causes and Controls* 3:77–81.

Hill, M J., and V. C Aries. 1971. Faecal steroid composition and its relationship to cancer of the large bowel. *Journal of Pathology* 104:129–139.

Hursting, S. D., S. N. Perkins, and J. M. Phang. 1994. Calorie restriction suppresses spontaneous tumorigenesis in p53-knockout transgenic mice. *Proceedings of the American Association of Cancer Research* 54:105.

Kato, I., S. Tominaga, Y. Ito, S. Kobayashi, Y. Yoshii, and A. Matsuura, et al. 1990. A comparative case-control analysis of stomach cancer and atrophic gastritis. *Cancer Research* 50:6559–6564.

Kneller, R. W., J. K. McLaughlin, E. Bjelke, L. M. Schuman, W. J. Blot, S. Wacholder, et al. 1991. A cohort study of stomach cancer in a high-risk American population. *Cancer* 68:672–678.

Kono, S., M. Ikeda, S. Tokudome, and M. Kuratsune. 1988. A case-control study of gastric cancer and diet in northern Kyushu, Japan. *Japanese Journal of Cancer Research* 79:1067–1074.

Kritchevsky, E., and D. M. Klurfeld. 1987. Caloric effects in experimental mammary tumorigenesis. *American Journal of Clinical Nutrition* 45(Suppl):236-242.

Kruis, W., G. Forstmaier, C. Sheurlen, and F. Stellard. 1991. Effect of diets low and high in refined sugars on gut transit, bile acid metabolism and bacterial fermentation. *Gut* 32:367–371.

Kuhnlein, H. V., D. H. Calloway, and B. F. Harland. 1979. Composition of traditional Hopi foods. *Journal of the American Dietetic Association* 75:37–41.

Kunitz, S. J., J. E. Levy, C. L. Odoroff, and J. Bollinger. 1979. The epidemiology of alcoholic cirrhosis in two southwestern Indian tribes. In *Beliefs, behaviors and alcoholic beverages: A cross–cultural survey,* ed. M. Marshall, 145–158. Ann Arbor: University of Michigan.

LaVecchia, C., A. Franceschi, P. Dolora, E. Bidoli, and F. Barbone. 1993. Refined sugar intake and the risk of colorectal cancer in humans. *International Journal of Cancer* 55:386–389.

LaVecchia, C., E. Negri, A. Decarli, et al. 1988. A case-control study of diet and colo-rectal cancer in northern Italy. *International Journal of Cancer* 41:492–498.

Lu, S. H., S. X. Chui, W. X Yang, X. N. Hu, L. P. Guo, and F. M. Li. 1991. Relevance of nitrosamines to esophageal cancer in China. *IARC Scientific Publications* 105:11–17.

May, P. A. 1982. Substance abuse and American Indians: Prevalence and susceptibility. *International Journal of Addiction* 17:1185–1209.

May, P. A., K. J. Hymbaugh, J. M. Aase, and J. M. Samet. 1983. Epidemiology of fetal alcohol syndrome among American Indians of the Southwest. *Social Biology* 30:374–387.

Morris, D. L., R. W. Buechley, C. R. Key, and M. V. Morgan. 1978. Gallbladder disease and gallbladder cancer among American Indians in tricultural New Mexico. *Cancer* 42(5):2472–2477.

National Academy of Sciences (NAS), commissioned by the National Cancer Institute (NCI). 1982. *Diet, nutrition and cancer.* Washington, DC: National Academy Press.

Nomura, A., J. S. Grove, G. N. Stemmermann, and R. K. Severson. 1990. A prospective study of stomach cancer and its relation to diet, cigarettes, and alcohol consumption. *Cancer Research* 50:627–631.

Nutting, P. A., W. L. Freeman, D. R. Risser, S. D. Helgerson, R. Paisano, J. Hisnanick, S. K. Beaver, I. Peters, J. P. Carney, and M. A. Speers. 1993. Cancer incidence among American Indians and Alaska Natives, 1980 through 1987. *American Journal of Public Health* 83(11):1589–1598.

Pariza, M. W. 1987. Fat, calories, and mammary carcinogenesis: Net energy effects. *American Journal of Clinical Nutrition* 45(Suppl):261–263.

Peto, R., R. Doll, J. D. Buckley, and M. D. Sporn. 1981. Can dietary beta-carotene materially reduce human cancer rates? *Nature* 290:201–208.

Poirier, L. A., P. M. Newberne, and M. W. Pariza, eds. 1986. *Essential nutrients in carcinogenesis.* New York: Plenum Press.

Potter, J. D., and A. J. McMichael. 1986. Diet and cancer of the colon and rectum: A case-control study. *Journal of the National Cancer Institute* 76:557–569.

Rohan, T. E., G. R. Howe, J. D. Burch, and M. Jain. 1995. Dietary factors and risk of prostate cancer: A case-control study in Ontario, Canada. *Cancer Causes and Controls* 6:145–154.

Sievers, M. L., and J. R. Fisher. 1983. Cancer in North American Indians: Environment versus heredity. *American Journal of Public Health* 73(5):485–487.

Smith, C. J., E. M. Manahan, S. G. Pablo. 1994. Food habit and cultural changes among the Pima Indians. In *Diabetes as a disease of civilization: The impact of culture change on indigenous peoples,* ed. J. R. Joe and R. S. Young, 407–433. New York: Mouton de Gruyter.

Smith, C. J., R. G. Nelson, H. R. Baird, S. A. Hardy, E. M. Manahan, P. H. Bennett, and W. C. Knowler. 1993. A survey of the dietary intake of the Pima Indians. Unpublished report supported in part by an NIH contract from the National Institute of Diabetes and Digestive and Kidney Diseases.

Sorem, K. A. 1985. Cancer incidence in the Zuni Indians of New Mexico. *Yale Journal of Biology and Medicine* 58:489–496.

Tannenbaum, A. 1959. Nutrition and cancer. In *The Physiopathology of Cancer,* ed. F. Homburger, 517–562. New York: Hoeber-Harper.

Teufel, N. I. 1989. Energy balance, obesity and acculturation among Hualapai Indian women of Arizona. Ph.D. Dissertation, University of Colorado.

—. 1994. Alcohol consumption and its effect on the dietary patterns of Hualapai Indian women. *Medical Anthropology* 16:79–97.

—. 1997. Development of culturally competent food-frequency questionnaires. *American Journal of Clinical Nutrition* 65(4):1173S–1178S.

—. 1998. Assessing diet-cancer associations in Native Americans. NCI-supported research in progress.

—. 1999. Nutritional problems of Native Americans. In *Primary care of Native American patients: Diagnosis, therapy, and epidemiology,* ed. J. M. Galloway, B. W. Goldberg, and J. S. Alpert, 283–292. Woburn, MA: Butterworth and Heinemann.

Teufel, N. I., and D. L. Dufour. 1990. Patterns of food use and nutrient intake of obese and non-obese Hualapai Indian women of Arizona. *Journal of the American Dietetic Association* 90(9):1229–1235.

Topper, M. D. 1980. Drinking as an expression of status: Navajo male adolescents. In *Drinking behavior among Southwestern Indians: An anthropological perspective,* ed. J. O. Waddell and M. W. Everett, 103–147. Tucson: University of Arizona Press.

Waddell, J. O., and M. W. Everett, eds. 1980. *Drinking behavior among southwestern Indians: An anthropological perspective.* Tucson: University of Arizona Press.

Wattenberg, L. W. 1983. Inhibition of neoplasia by minor dietary constituents. *Cancer Research* 43(Suppl):2448S–2453S.

—. 1992. Inhibition of carcinogenesis by minor dietary constituents. *Cancer Research* 52(Suppl):2085S–2091S.

WCRF/AICR. 1997. *Food, nutrition and the prevention of cancer: A global perspective.* Washington, DC: World Cancer Research Fund/American Institute for Cancer Research.

Wolfe, W. S., C. W. Weber, and K. D. Arviso. 1985. Use and nutrient composition of traditional Navajo foods. *Ecology of Food and Nutrition* 17:323–344.

Yu, G. P., C. C. Hsieh, L. Y. Wang, S. Z. Yu, X. L. Li, and T. H. Jin. 1995. Green-tea consumption and risk of stomach cancer: A population-based case-control study in Shanghai, China. *Cancer Causes and Controls* 6:532–538.

Zheng, T., P. Boyle, W. C. Willett, H. Hu, J. Dan, et al. 1992. A case-control study of oral cancer in Bejing, People's Republic of China: Associations with nutrient intakes, foods, and food groups. *European Journal of Cancer* 29B:45–55.

Table 15.1
Dietary–Cancer Association [1]

Cancer Site	*Increased (8) or Decreased (9) Incidence in Southwest Native Americans as Compared to U.S., All Races[2]*	*Dietary Risk Factors*	*Nondietary Factors*
Breast[3]	9	Low intake of vegetables High intake of alcohol High prevalence of obesity	Rapid early growth Early menarche
Endometrium[3]	9	High prevalence of obesity	Nulliparity
Cervix	8	Low intake of fruits and vegetables	High prevalence of HPV High prevalence of smoking
Colon, rectum[3]	9	Low intake of vegetables High intake of meat, especially grilled, barbecued, cured, and fried High intake of eggs High intake of alcohol High body mass index	Low physical activity
Esophagus[3]	9	Low intake of fruits and vegetables High intake of alcohol	High prevalence of smoking
Gallbladder[3]	8	High body mass index	
Liver	8	High intake of alcohol High intake of contaminated food	
Lung[3]	9	Low intake of fruits and vegetables	High prevalence of smoking
Mouth, Pharynx, Nasopharnyx, Larnyx[3]	9	Low intake of fruits and vegetables High intake of salted fish High intake of alcohol	High prevalence of smoking and chewing tobacco
Pancreas	9	Low intake of fruits and vegetables High intake of meat High intake of animal fat High intake of energy	High prevalence of smoking
Prostate	9	High intake of meat High intake of animal fat High intake of dietary fat	
Stomach	8	Low intake of fruits and vegetables	High prevalence of HPV

Table 15.1 Dietary–Cancer Association [1]			
		High intake of grilled and barbecued meats Low intake of whole grains High intake of salt or salted foods Low intake of tea (green) Poor access to refrigeration	

Notes:

1. Associations listed as "probable" or "possible" by the World Cancer Research Fund and the American Institute of Clinical Research (WCRF/AICR 1997).

2. Indicates that proposed diet-cancer associations are not supported by correlation or ecologic studies among Southwest Native Americans.

3. Comparative incidence data drawn from Baquet et al. (1992); Burhansstipanov and Dresser (1993); Nutting et al. (1993); and Sorem (1985).

Table 15.2 Dietary Carcinogens Associated with Food Handling, Preparation, and Storage	
Dietary Carcinogens	*Association with Food*
Aflatoxins	Found in moldy foods
Heterocyclic amines	Found in meat cooked at very high temperatures
N-nitroso compounds	Found in some spoiled foods, some dried foods, and some high protein foods
Polycyclic aromatic hydrocarbons	Products of combustion; found in cooked foods and dark beer

Table 15.3
Dietary Characteristics Associated with Increased Cancer Risk

Dietary Characteristics	*Proposed Mechanism of Increased Cancer Risk*
High energy (calorie) intake	Supports cell proliferation
High fat intake	Supports cell proliferation Stimulates excretion of bile acid in the gut
High animal protein intake (includes eggs)	Supports cell proliferation
High refined carbohydrate/sugar intake	Supports cell proliferation, possibly by elevating plasma glucose and insulin levels Slows gut transit time, increasing contact time between mucosa and carcinogens in gastro-intestinal tract Stimulates high bile excretion; bile acid may be carcinogenic, particularly to colon cells
High alcohol intake	May alter mucosal cells of upper respiratory and digestive tract Induces micronutrient dietary deficiencies Damages liver cells Influences estrogen levels
High intake of salt, and salted, cured, pickled, and smoked meats and fish	Damages gastric mucosa May contain carcinogenic N-nitroso compounds
High intake of grilled and barbecued meats	May contain heterocyclic amines
High meal frequency	Promotes bile acid excretion and gastro-ileal reflex Increases chance of contact between potentially carcinogenic bile acids and colon cells

Table 15.4
Dietary Components Associated with Reduced Cancer Risk

Dietary Component	*Proposed Mechanism of Cancer Protection*
VITAMINS	
Carotenoids	• Antioxidant capabilities • Supports immune function • Supports normal cell growth, maintenance, and differentiation
Vitamin C	• Antioxidant capabilities • Supports immune function
Vitamin E	• Antioxidant capabilities • Supports immune function
Folate	• Essential to normal DNA replication
MINERALS	
Selenium	• Enhances immune function • Decreases mutagenic effect of carcinogens • Suppresses cancer cell proliferation
DIETARY FIBER	
	• Dilutes of carcinogenic agents • Promotes carcinogen elimination, reducing tissue-carcinogen contact
BIOACTIVE COMPOUNDS	
Protease inhibitors	• Blocks enzyme activity associated with invasive capacity of cancer cells
Flavonoids	• Antioxidant capabilities
Terpenoids (specifically limonene)	• Induces enzyme activity associated with cancer protection
Isoflavones and lignans	• Acts as phytoestrogens, binding to estrogen receptors and blocking activity of potentially carcinogenic estrogens
Polyphenols (green tea extract)	• Inhibits carcinogenesis in cells of digestive tract

Table 15.5

Anthropometric and Dietary Characteristics of Native American Women Representing Four Tribes of the Southwestern United States

TRIBE (N)	Hualapai[1] (N=28)	Apache [2] (N=27)	Pima [3] (N=273)	Navajo [4] (N=225)	Target Ranges[5]
ANTHROPOMETRIC DATA					
Age range [6]	18-35	16-76	18-74	20-39	≥ 18
BMI (kg/m^2)	31.0+4.[7]	NR	33.7±6.8	28.7±0.4	18.5-25
DIETARY INTAKES[8]					
Total Fat (% kcal)	35.0	35.3	36.2	35	15-30
Carbohydrate (% kcal)	52.5	49.1	48.5	49	55-75
Protein (% kcal)	12.5	14.3	15.7	16	9-12
Alcohol (% kcal)	5.1	*1.8* [9]	*0.3*	NR	<2.5
Dietary Fiber (gm/day)	4.4±2.0	5.0±1.1	*23.5±0.9*	14±1	20-35
SELECT VITAMIN AND MICRONUTRIENT INTAKES					
Folate (µg/day)	249±113	206±93.4	NR	220±15	250-450
Vitamin C (mg/day)	79.5±58.2	63.0±40.5	98.7±6.9	95±10	175-400
Beta-Caro[10] (µg RE/day)	243.9± 134.2	107±78.1	1991±238	341±52	9000-18000
Vitamin E (µg/day)	*9.7±3.6*	*6.37±4.14*	NR	*7.1±0.8*	4-7
FRUIT AND VEGETABLE INTAKES					
Fruits/ Veges (serv/day)	0.45±0.81	0.46± 0.75	NR	< 1.0	5.0-10.0

NOTES

1.   Seven twenty-four-hour dietary recalls collected from twenty-eight women (De Giovanni 1995; Teufel 1989; Teufel and Dufour 1990).

2.   Six twenty-four-hour recalls collected from twenty-seven women (De Giovanni 1995; Teufel 1997).

3.   One twenty-four-hour dietary recall collected from 273 women (Smith et al. 1993).

4.   One twenty-four-hour dietary recall collected from 225 women (Ballew et al. 1997).

5.   Target ranges for nutrient intakes were derived from the recommendations of the World Cancer Research Fund and American Institute for Cancer Research Report (WCRF/AICR 1997).

6.   Age range is provided, as not all reports provided mean age.

7.   NR = not reported.

8.   Macronutrient distribution represented as a percentage of total energy intake.

9.   Bolded and italicized mean intakes indicate that mean intake fell within the range recommended by the WCRF/AICR.

10.   Beta-Caro stands for beta-carotene which is a cartenoid and a vitamin A compound.

Concluding Remarks

John Molina and Diane Weiner

This book presents the multiple ways in which people, both lay and professional, create and enact their own cultures, and subcultures, of cancer. These cultures must not be perceived as stereotypical phenomena—stuck in time or attributed to members of a "quaint" community. The cultures of cancer are continuously changing and evolving, framed by individual and group histories, social networks, technologies, politics, economics, religions, and other factors that serve as environmental forces.

Most importantly, there are observed differences in thought and practice between and among "like groups of people," such as doctors, holistic practitioners, or members of ethnic groups. Although oncologists may undergo similar types of training and may encounter similar types of problems, they interpret situations and develop coping and negotiating strategies in ways that are shaped by, but not solely determined by, their respective education, occupation, or status. A patient and members of his/her support network may move toward acceptance of cancer by placing it into a framework that fits his/her cultural system (see also Garro 1990; Hunt, in this volume). Only then can total well-being be achieved in a physiological, psychosocial, or spiritual sense. The contributors to this volume demonstrate that there exists a variety of perceptions about prevention and control as well as myriad ways to approach these complex concepts and processes. The meanings of prevention and control may be quite diverse. Lay people not only may have understandings different from those of doctors and researchers but occasionally challenge research agendas and regulatory policies; they very frequently seek alternative and complementary cancer therapies in order to obtain efficacious care.

The authors who contributed to Part I, Cancer Beliefs and Behaviors, demonstrate that most people need and look for solutions to health problems that enable them to interpret and act on conditions of health and illness that are linked to life experiences and relationships and their own spirituality (see also Kleinman 1988; Steptoe et al. 1991; Holland 1996; Ferrell et al. 1998; Montbriand 1998).

In Part II, Interventions in Review, we find that while some cancers may have a lower incidence rate among an ethnic or racial group, survival rates may be extremely poor. Contributors reflect on projects that target specific populations, in order to address issues of cancer screening, environmental exposure, and cancer treatment availability. What makes interventions advantageous? How can success be defined? Is achievement measured by increased participation in a clinical trial, by satisfied and meaningful involvement in that trial, or by financial standards set by its administrators? Perhaps success can be measured by the opportunity for individuals to decrease the incidence of cancer mortality. If so, we must identify what enhances the ability of programs to succeed.

Motivation to participate in a screening or a treatment is based not solely on some behavioral health model but also on the ability of guides, whether they be professionals or lay "experts," to explain consistently the objectives and methods of a program, protocol, or lesson in a sensitive or culturally competent manner, and to respond to participants' questions, needs, and concerns. Trust, faith, and empathy aid in the establishment of a meaningful relationship. These values frequently originate in active participation of community members as creators or managers of, advisers to, or advocates of programs.

In other cases, practitioners and scholars may demean or negate the lay etiological beliefs attached to prevention practices (see Chavez et al. 1995; Modiano 1995). Such intellectual chauvinism and discrimination may deter lay people from seeking clinical assistance. As Kagawa-Singer and Maxwell assert, it may be more beneficial to stress or elaborate upon lay etiological beliefs linked to effective detection and treatment practices rather than to try and dispel these ideas. It is not important that the practitioner believe what the patient believes; it is imperative that the views of the patient be noted, clarified, and valued by providers, administrators, and policy makers. This acknowledgment should provide enhanced comprehension by lay people of medical ideas (see Julia 1996). Innovations perceived to be useful by clients, especially those that do not subvert religious or philosophical beliefs, may thus be more likely to be accepted (see Adair et al. 1988).

One way to create a foundation for flexible interventions is to obtain sound empirical data on a subject. The National Cancer Institute suggests that the

strongest evidence [of a prevention strategy] would be that obtained from a well-designed and well-conducted randomized controlled trial with cancer specific mortality as the endpoint. It is, however, not always practical to conduct such a trial to address every question in the field of cancer prevention (National Cancer Institute 1998, 1).

The National Cancer Institute describes other types of research, all of which tend clinically, ecologically, or epidemiologically to address the examination of large populations (National Cancer Institute 1998). In Part III, New Strategies for Cancer Research, a health educator, Burhansstipanov, and two anthropologists,

Staten and Teufel, examine innovative research topics in distinct ways. They all dispel the myth of a single hegemonic science of cancer. Laura Nader asserts that

the boundaries of science are drawn and redrawn. Borders are contentious, and as any scientist knows, science is not a revealed and unambiguous truth—today's science may be tomorrow's pseudoscience or vice versa.

What is at issue is whether a narrowly demarcated science—one restricted to contemporary western ways of knowing—provides us with the greatest source of truth. (Nader 1996, 3)

This stance is not meant to invalidate the work of clinical, ecologic, or epidemiologic studies; rather, Nader suggests that other methodologies, or ways of knowing, may also have validity (see also Martin 1994; Ritenbaugh 1995; Claeson et al. 1996).

Obviously, a plethora of creative research styles exist. For the authors in this volume, the objective is to employ methodologies that explore and enable indigenous knowledge systems by utilizing a community-based approach. By indigenous we mean native to a group, whether the membership is composed of molecular geneticists from a university, apple farmers in rural Washington, or Hmong housewives of Long Beach, California. Carefully analyzed data can then be used to develop and implement personalized or group interventions that address the health needs and priorities of a person or community in a modality that fits the cultural belief system. Therein lies the success of any intervention program.

RESEARCH IMPLICATIONS

Several types of research are needed. Our suggestions encompass merely a few topics. Epidemiological data and quality of life data concerning cancer survivors is lacking. Who survives, and why? We find that stage of disease and treatment modalities do not always predict cancer survival rates. Factors that appear to influence outcome, but that have not been thoroughly studied, include social support systems and spirituality.

Hunt writes that the biomedical model carries great social authority and technical promise. She argues that medical explanations are seldom rejected. When, how, and why are they forsaken? Are they abandoned only if a cancer is considered to be incurable? What roles do individual and family histories and stories play in this situation?

The biomedical model attributes cancer to a biological process. Often there is little or no regard for the psychosocial aspect of a patient's response to a threat to life or a possibility there of (see also Montbriand 1998). The patient may accept the medical diagnosis and treatment, but the illness introduces a complete disruption in the physical, social, and emotional state of the patient. This illness is thus difficult to integrate into belief systems, which are distinct from biomedical systems. Conflict produces psychological and mental distress that may impact the course of treatment and eventual medical outcome. We must learn more about the ways in which clients, members of their support systems, and their health professionals can possibly reduce and alleviate strife.

Emotional tension is often mediated by expressions of religious activity. What can examinations of religious beliefs and behaviors—whether they be Charismatic Christian, Muslim, Buddhist, or other—teach about the cancer prevention and control attitudes and actions of believers? Personal religious beliefs are important in helping patients contend with diagnoses of cancer. Religion and spirituality may enable an individual to find a personal meaning as well as the emotional strength to cope with illness (Hassey Dow et al. 1996; Ferrell et al. 1998). What are the ways, if any, in which providers, administrators, or health educators might enhance opportunities for religious and spiritual activities, if desired by clients?

Continued explorations of providers, including their expectations, communication approaches, and processes of negotiation, are quite necessary (see also Ritenbaugh 1995). We need to clarify the social, emotional, and spiritual perspectives and motivations of different practitioners. Balshem provides an extremely useful start for continued studies of oncologists. A patient of Dr. Molina's recently died at home with a recurrence of pancreatic cancer. On the evening before she died, Dr. Molina visited her:

I held her hand. She looked at me during her waking moments—she had a morphine drip—and smiled. She was not afraid or sad, but happy. Her spirituality was evident by the crosses hanging on her bed, a picture of Jesus and the Virgin Mary on her wall. But the success of that spirituality was noted by the smile on her face as she said to me, "I am ready to go. . . . Thank you for helping me. . . ." Before I left, I prayed with her. I am Protestant. She is Catholic. But there is no distinction in spiritual matters. She died the next morning.

An oncologist, like other providers, needs to find his/her own spirituality that will aid his/her patients' experiences of death and distress. This spirituality will help patients and their families through the most difficult moments. As Dr. Molina was once told by an oncologist, "We not only help people live—we help them die when it is their time." It would be wise for us to learn more about the coping strategies of oncologists.

Traditional healers, medicine men and women, and *curanderos* and *curanderas* have for centuries provided the medical care and healing in their communities. These practitioners still exist and offer healing ceremonies and various types of traditional medicine, herbs, rituals, and manipulations for ill individuals and their families. For many people this type of intervention is important in cases of cancer, because the etiology may appear to be unclear or mysterious, and the psyche of the person and members of his/her support network may be disturbed by the illness. The traditional healer aids a patient in the understanding of the illness (see Kleinman 1980; Hahn 1995; Molina 1997). Understanding an etiology may also help a patient (and his/her family members) rest an "unsettled psyche" and promote a positive attitude toward working with an oncologist or other health professional.

If we want to make an impact on the health status of any population, we must identify not only the major genetic causes but also the social, behavioral and environmental factors associated with morbidity and mortality. In his practice, Dr. Molina sees many Hispanics whose lifestyles include rigorous labor (landscaping, construction, housekeeping) and whose lack of transportation makes them pedestrians. As Staten reveals in her chapter, these high levels of activity may be excluded from typical "exercise" assessment tools. In retrospect, these aspects of lifestyle may be deemed healthy in terms of cancer prevention, yet they may be unacknowledged in research. How might other ethnic/racial, economic, age, occupational, or other populations define and express behaviors that may influence health status? What are the physical activities of Russian immigrants in New York? What might an Appalachian woman believe is a "good" or "healthy" exercise program? Does she even use such a framework? If so, how might she behave in accordance with such perceptions? Epidemiologic studies of lay etiologies would increase our understanding of such concepts (Ritenbaugh 1995).

It is essential to devise projects that investigate the social dynamics of prevention, control, and healing in order to facilitate screening programs among those who feel that they are not ill. For example, we need more in-depth investigations of the reasons women who claim to know breast self-exam techniques do not use them (see Lanier and Kelly). Why are women afraid of what they might find? Why is this fear more profound than fear of the possibility of death? These types of projects or screenings may have to evaluate issues pertinent to a person and her family. What are the "guiding principles" in her life? For what and whom does she and her family live?

Screening programs look for disease in people who feel "well." It may be that knowledge of having a disease decreases participation in a screening program. This knowledge will disrupt lives and result in subsequent evaluations and treatments that the individual may not be psychologically, nor even financially, equipped to handle. This may be especially true if a person feels that the findings of an "early cancer" will impose hardships on family members. Indeed, most diseases tend to be incidental findings or in later symptomatic stages, which accounts for the higher morbidity rates of cancer as noted by many of the authors. The way to increase utilization of screening programs may be intervention projects that focus on education rather than on the disease itself. Lanier and Kelly found an association between knowledge and behavior. The higher the knowledge score, the less likely a person was to be in a high-risk category for health behaviors. A potentially successful intervention could include education on the clinical perspective of the disease process itself; etiology, treatments, outcomes; and success stories of other survivors. Town meetings, group discussions, and secular talking circles are excellent social environments, which offer comfort and safety. Fear of the unknown may be dispelled. Knowledge of a disease, with at least some consternation alleviated, may increase acceptability of a screening test, whether it be a self-exam or a clinical exam.

PRACTICAL IMPLICATIONS

Even though prevention and treatment programs frequently focus on individuals, they rarely act alone when pursuing health care objectives (see also Kleinman et al. 1992; Hahn 1995). Those seeking information or screening (the undiagnosed and the well), patients, and lay caregivers tend to share experiences with a variety of social support network members—both lay and professional. Health care providers of distinct types (clinical, clerical, alternative, tribal, folk, and divinely inspired) often share healing responsibilities with colleagues and with those who use different techniques. In some cases, providers from distinct health care traditions attempt to work cooperatively, while other practitioners may be unaware of others' attempts or may act in contradiction to them. Clients must have the chance to work with different types of caregivers, whether they be herbalists, acupuncturists, or oncologists, if clients so choose. Ideally, practitioners should also have the opportunity to operate in a cooperative and multidisciplinary mode.

Balshem asks how medical expertise and authority can be reshaped in order to enhance cancer prevention and control. One way is to provide practitioners of different approaches with intellectual interactions. The time available to most practicing clinicians is severely limited; classes and university research settings may prove useful for such encounters. For example, oncology students might benefit from even limited training sessions with local herbalists. Moreover, herbalists would learn more about oncological perspectives. In later years, patients may utilize both providers.

Hess (1997) argues that breast cancer patients want "sophisticated, well-informed, open-minded clinicians who would serve as a mentor and a teacher to help guide an individually tailored combination of the best of biomedical and ACCT" cancer treatments. Patients may desire or demand integrated programs of psychospiritual, nutritional/metabolic, exercise, and destressing interventions (see also Montbriand 1998). These approaches offer ways to obtain "calibrated, achievable and realistic bits" of hope in terms of healing (Good et al. 1990, 72). These methods may truly reorient "medical expertise and authority" thereby increasing an individual and communal sense of empowerment.

Indeed, people want to know about health care programs and options. Leaders of ACCTs, recent immigrants to the United States, office workers, and others seek understandable information. In a recent ethnographic study, more than seventy people interviewed requested additional information on cancer (Weiner 1997). When asked what they might like to learn more about, questions included: "If my grandfather and father had prostate cancer, what chance do I have to get prostate cancer?" "Is it true if a person has cancer and you open the body during surgery the cancer spreads, or is that a myth"? "What does cancer look like?" Clinicians need to ask their clients *and* members of their social networks: What do they want to know more about? Is there anything that needs to be made clearer? These inquiries may seem simple, but lay people are rarely asked these questions.

These type of cancer communication practices can engage and encourage people to be active participants in the healing process. Storytelling, support groups, formal education programs, videos, and practitioner-client interactions all should be viewed as possible teaching methods. It is crucial to avoid, as Green and Werner state, the mistake of "talking down to people." Hierarchical communication practices serve little purpose other than to marginalize the thoughts and behaviors of clients (Kuipers 1989; Borges and Waitzkin 1995). Misinterpretations and confusion on the parts of clients as well as providers may be the result (Davis 1993; Weiner in press). To minimize possible miscommunication, health education messages may have to be revised or created anew. Community participation in the development of these messages will eliminate a barrage of communication problems.

In a final note, we must tackle racial, ethnic, linguistic, religious, economic, and gender discrimination, whether in subtle or overt forms. Moore describes a few overt examples of prejudice; they represent dismal failures of the biomedical health system. Discrimination may also occur subtly. For example, providers and program administrators often use the term "fatalism" when they do not understand the actions of clients. This term is generally attached to the actions of "Others"—people distinct from the educational, economic, or social classes of those who use this term. Fatalism implies inaction—a giving into the "Fates." Certain people may indeed be labeled fatalists, but as we see in many of the chapters of this book, people are also decision makers. However, they may take different courses of action, with distinct time frames, than health professionals expect. Ideas of fatalism do indeed exist; the term, however, seems to be overused.

Most acts of discrimination toward cancer patients, or within the health care system in general, that exclude the plethora of worthy data on economic discrimination, are not discussed as major parts of the problem of cancer prevention and control (for recent research on this topic see Lannin et al. 1998). This situation has to be rectified, or psychosocial and physiological distress as well as disparities in mortality are likely to continue (see also Dressler 1993; Harrison 1994; Trotman Reid 1994). Examinations of the loci of structural power are needed. We must also investigate what other discriminatory acts take place consciously or subconsciously, and who the perpetrators are of such acts. Such inquiries need not be limited to empirical research. They should also involve individual self reviews—the first steps toward real change.

This text centers on the social, cultural, and behavioral aspects of cancer prevention and control. It is merely a beginning. We must continue to examine not only the bodies but the emotions, spirits, and thoughts of individuals.

LITERATURE CITED

Adair, J., K. Deuschle, and C. Barnett. 1988. *The people's health: Anthropology and medicine in Navajo society.* Albuquerque: University of New Mexico Press.
Borges, S. and H. Waitzkin. 1995. Women's narratives in primary care medical encounters. *Women and Health* 23(1):29–55.
Chavez, L., F. A. Hubbard, J. M. McMullin, R. G. Martinez, and S. I. Mishra. 1995. Structure and meaning in models of breast and cervical cancer risk factors: A compari-

226   Concluding Remarks

son of perceptions among Latinas, Anglo women, and physicians. *Medical Anthropology Quarterly* 9(1):40–74.

Claeson, B., E. Martin, W. Richardson, M. Schoch-Spana, and K. Taussig. 1996. Scientific literacy, what it is, why it's important, and why scientists think we don't have it: The case of immunology and the immune system. In *Naked science: Anthropological inquiry into boundaries, power, and knowledge*. ed. Laura Nader, 101–116. New York: Routledge.

Davis, K. 1993. Nice doctors and invisible patients: The problem of power in feminist common sense. In *The social organization of doctor-patient communication*, ed. Alexandra Dundas Todd and Sue Fisher, 243–265. Norwood, NJ: Ablex.

Dressler, W. W. 1993. Health in the African American community: Accounting for health inequalities. *Medical Anthropology Quarterly* 7(4):325–346.

Ferrell, B. R., M. Grant, B. Funk, S. Otis-Green, and N. Garcia. 1998. Quality of life in breast cancer: Part II: Psychological and spiritual well-being. *Cancer Nursing* 21(1):1–9.

Garro, L. C. 1990. Continuity and change: The interpretation of illness in an Anishinaabe (Ojibway) community. *Culture, Medicine, and Psychiatry* 14:417–454.

Good, M. J. D., B. J. Good, C. Schaffer, and S. E. Lind. 1990. American oncology and the discourse on hope. *Culture, Medicine, and Psychiatry* 14:59–79.

Hahn, R. A. 1995. *Sickness and healing: An anthropological perspective*. New Haven, CT: Yale University Press.

Harrison, F. V. 1994. Racial and gender inequalities in health and health care. *Medical Anthropology Quarterly* 8(1):90–95.

Hassey Dow, K., B. R. Ferrell, S. Leigh, J. Ly, and P. Gulasekaram. 1996. An evaluation of the QQL among long-term survivors of breast cancer. *Breast Cancer Research and Treatment* 39:261–273.

Hess, D. 1997. Personal communication.

Holland, J. 1996. Cancer's psychological challenges. *Scientific American* 275(3):158–161.

Julia, M. C., ed. 1996. *Multicultural awareness in the health care professions*. Boston: Allyn and Bacon.

Kleinman, A. 1980. *Patients and healers in the context of culture*. Berkeley: University of California Press.

—. 1988. *The illness narratives: Suffering, healing, and the human condition*. New York: Basic Books.

Kleinman, A., P. E. Brodwin, B. J. Good, M. J. D. Good. 1992. Pain as human experience: An introduction. In *Pain as human experience: An anthropological perspective*, ed. Mary-Jo DelVecchio Good, Paul E. Brodwin, Byron J. Good, and Arthur Kleinman, 1–28. Berkeley: University of California Press.

Kuipers, J. 1989. "Medical discourse" in anthropological context: Views of language and power. *Medical Anthropology Quarterly* 3(2):99–123.

Lannin, Donald R., Holly F. Mathews, Jim Mitchell, Melvin S. Swanson, Frances H. Swanson, and Maxine S. Edwards. 1998. Influence of socioeconomic and cultural factors on racial differences in late-stage presentation of breast cancer. *Journal of the American Medical Association* 279 (22):1801–1807.

Martin, E. 1994. *Flexible bodies: The role of immunity in American culture from the days of polio to the age of AIDS*. Boston: Beacon.

Modiano, M. R. 1995. Breast and cervical cancer in Hispanic women. *Medical Anthropology Quarterly* 9(1):75–76.

Molina, J. 1997. Cultural medicine. *Journal for Minority Medical Students* (Spring):28–32.

Montbriand, Muriel. 1998. Abandoning biomedicine for alternate therapies: Oncology patients' stories. *Cancer Nursing* 21(1):36–45.

Nader, Laura. 1996. Introduction: Anthropological inquiry into boundaries, power, and knowledge. In *Naked Science: Anthropological inquiry into boundaries, power, and knowledge.* ed. Laura Nader, 1–29. New York: Routledge.

National Cancer Institute. 1997. Cancer facts: Highlights of NCI's prevention and control programs.

—.1998. PDQ supportive care/screening/prevention information. http://www.ncc.go/jp/cnet/htm/. Accessed: July 1998.

Ritenbaugh, C. 1995. Commentary on "models of cancer risk factors." *Medical Anthropology Quarterly* 9(1):77–79.

Steptoe, A., I. Sutcliffe, B. Allen, and C. Coombes. 1991. Satisfaction with communication, medical knowledge, and coping style in patients with metastatic cancer. *Social Science and Medicine* 32(6):627–632

Trotman Reid, P. 1994. Identifying racism is necessary but not sufficient for the future. *Medical Anthropology Quarterly* 8(1):100–101.

Weiner, D. In press. Ethnogenetics: Interpreting ideas about diabetes and inheritance. *American Indian Culture and Research Journal.*

—. 1997. *Southern California Indian cancer prevention: Belief systems, support networks, and treatments,* field notes.

Selected Bibliography

Balshem, M. 1993. *Cancer in the community: Class and medical authority.* Washington, DC: Smithsonian Institution Press.

Bastani, R., A. Marcus, A. Maxwell, I. P. Das, and K. X. Yan. 1994. Evaluation of an intervention to increase mammography screening in Los Angeles. *Preventive Medicine* 23:83–90.

Burhansstipanov, L. 1997. *Cancer among elder Native Americans.* Denver: University of Colorado, Health Sciences Center, National Center for American Indian and Alaska Native Mental Health Research.

Cassileth, B. R., and C. C. Chapman. 1996. Alternative and complementary cancer therapies. *Cancer* 77(6):1026–1033.

Chavez, L., A. Hubbell, J. McMullin, R. Martinez, and S. Mishra. 1995. Understanding knowledge and attitudes about breast cancer: A cultural analysis. *Archives of Family Medicine* 4:145–152.

Davis, S. M. 1994. General guidelines for an effective and culturally sensitive approach to health education. In *The multicultural challenge in health education,* ed. A. C. Matiella, 117–132. Santa Cruz, CA: ETR Associates.

Doll, R., and R. Peto. 1981. The causes of cancer: Quantitative estimates of avoidable risks of cancer in the United States today. *Journal of the National Cancer Institute* 66:1191–1308.

Glover, Claudia Sanchez, and Felicia Schanche Hodge, eds. *Native outreach—A report to American Indian, Alaska Native, and Native Hawaiian communities.* NIH Pub. No. 98–4341. Bethesda, MD: National Cancer Institute.

Good, M. J. D., B. J. Good, C. Schaffer and S. E. Lind. 1990. American oncology and the discourse on hope. *Culture, Medicine, and Psychiatry* 14(1):59–79.

Haynes, M. Alfred, and Brian D. Smedley, eds. 1999. *The unequal burden of cancer: An asssessment of NIH research and programs for ethnic minorities and the medically underserved.* Washington, DC: National Academy Press.

Hess, D. 1997. *Can bacteria cause cancer? Alternative medicine confronts big science.*

New York: New York University Press.

—1999. *Evaluating alternative cancer therapies: A guide to the science and politics of an emerging medical field*. New Brunswick, NJ: Rutgers University Press.

Hodge, F. S., L. Fredericks, and B. Rodriguez. 1996. American Indian women's talking circle: A cervical cancer screening and prevention project. *Cancer* Supp 78(7):1592–1597.

Hunt, L. M. 1998. Moral reasoning and the meaning of cancer: Causal explanations of oncologists and patients in southern Mexico. *Medical Anthropology Quarterly* 12(3):298–318.

Kagawa-Singer, M. 1997. Addressing issues for early detection and screening in ethnic populations. *Oncology Nursing Forum* 24:1705–1714.

Marcus, A., and L. Crane. 1998. A review of cervical cancer screening intervention research: Implications for public health programs and future research. *Preventive Medicine* 27(1):13–31.

Miller, B. A. et al., eds. 1996. *Racial/ethnic patterns of cancer in the United States 1988-1992*. NIH Pub. No. 96–4104. Bethesda: National Cancer Institute.

Morra, M., and E. Potts. 1994. *Choices*. New York: Avon Books.

Moss, R. 1996. *The cancer industry*. Brooklyn, NY: Equinox.

Needham, C. 1994. Cultural differences shape cancer care. *Journal of National Cancer Institute* 86(4):261–262.

Pasick, J., et al. 1996. Similarities and differences across cultures: Questions to inform a third generation for health promotion. *Health Education Quarterly* 23 Supp:142–161.

Spiegel, D. 1997. Psychosocial aspects of breast cancer treatment. *Seminars in Oncology* 24(1)S1:36–47.

Tannock, I. F., and R. Hill. 1998. *The basic science of oncology*. 3d ed.Toronto: Ontario Cancer Institute and University of Toronto.

Teufel, N. 1997. Development of culturally competent food frequency questionnaires. *American Journal of Clinical Nutrition* 65 Supp:1173S–1178S.

WCRF/AICR. 1997. *Food, nutrition and the prevention of cancer: A global perspective*. Washington, DC: World Cancer Research Fund/American Institute for Cancer Research.

Weinberg, Robert A. 1998. *One renegade cell: How cancer begins*. New York: Basic Books.

Wooddell, Margaret J., and David J. Hess. 1998. *Women confront cancer: Making medical history by choosing alternative and complementary therapies*. New York: New York University Press.

Index

About the Contributors

Bruce Allen, Jr., is an Assistant Professor in the Department of Obstetrics and Gynecology at Charles R. Drew University of Medicine and Science.

Martha Balshem is an Associate Professor in the University Studies Program at Portland State University.

Linda Burhansstipanov is the Director of the Native American Cancer Center of Excellence in Pine, Colorado.

Janice Allen Chilton is currently a Cancer Prevention Specialist and Study Coordinator for the Women's Healthy Eating and Living (WHEL) Study at the University of Texas M. D. Anderson Cancer Center.

Leslie Cunningham-Sabo is a Research Nutritionist and Health Educator at the Center for Health Promotion and Disease Prevention, University of New Mexico.

Sally M. Davis is Director of one of the Centers for Disease Control's Prevention Research Centers and is an Associate Professor of Pediatrics at the University of New Mexico School of Medicine.

Angelina Esparza is the Community Relations Coordinator for University of Texas M. D. Anderson Cancer Center.

Sarah Ann G. Garza is the Research Dietitian/Coordinator of The Kellogg's Hispanic Nutrition Intervention Study, Department of Gynecologic Oncology, University of Texas M. D. Anderson Cancer Center.

Rosie Gonzalez is the former Study Coordinator and head Dietitian for the Compañeras Sanas project.

Bettye Green is a nurse at Saint Joseph's Medical Center, South Bend, Indiana, the Educator for Community Outreach Programs, the Coordinator of the Hospital-Based School Nurse Program, and the Coordinator of the Parish Health Ministry.

Richard A. Hajek is a Research Scientist the University of Texas M. D. Anderson Cancer Center.

David J. Hess is an Associate Professor of Anthropology in the Sciences and Technology Studies Department, School of Humanities and Social Sciences, Rensselaer Polytechnic Institute.

Linda M. Hunt is an Associate Professor in the Department of Anthropology at Michigan State University.

Jennie R. Joe is a Professor in the Department of Family and Community Medicine and the Director of the Native American Research and Training Center at the University of Arizona.

Lovell A. Jones is a Professor and the Director of Experimental Gynecologic Oncology/Endocrinology at the University of Texas M. D. Anderson Cancer Center.

Marjorie Kagawa-Singer is an Assistant Professor at the UCLA School of Public Health and Asian American Studies Center, and is a Lecturer on the faculty of the School of Nursing.

Judith Kaur is an Assistant Professor of Oncology at the Mayo Medical School, Mayo Clinic, Rochester, Minnesota.

Janet J. Kelly is an epidemiologic consultant residing in Anchorage, Alaska.

Anne P. Lanier teaches at the University of Alaska, Anchorage and the University of Washington and is also the Director of the Arctic Investigation Laboratory and the Area Epidemiologist for Alaska Area Native Health Service.

Annette E. Maxwell is an Associate Researcher in Cancer Control at the UCLA Jonsson Comprehensive Cancer Center.

John Molina is the founder and director of Las Fuentes Health Clinic of Guadalupe, Guadalupe, Arizona and practices in the Department of Ambulatory Care and Community Health Services at the Phoenix Indian Medical Center.

Rhonda J. Moore is a Postdoctoral Fellow at the University of Texas M. D. Anderson Cancer Center.

Maria Rocio-Moguel is a a Nutritional Research Assistant at University of Texas M. D. Anderson Cancer Center.

Lisa K. Staten is a Research Assistant Professor of Public Health at the University of Arizona Health Sciences Center.

Nicolette I. Teufel is a Research Assistant Professor at the University of Arizona, Department of Preventive Medicine.

Diane Weiner is a Professional Research Anthropologist at the UCLA American Indian Studies Center.

Ellen Werner is a Senior Health Scientist at Temple University Institute for Survey Research.

A special credit goes to Ramsey Ellis and Keeli Tebeau for their computer assistance. Thanks to Jan Weiner and Lillian Weiner for editorial assistance.

ISBN 0-275-96180-X

90000>

HARDCOVER BAR CODE